LOBSTERS AS SENTINELS

Lobsters as Sentinels

Monitoring Coastal Ecosystem Health

SANYUB S.

Spectra Enterprise

CONTENTS

INDEX

INTRODUCTION

Beach front environments, with their unpredictable embroidery of life and dynamic connections, stand as fundamental marks of our planet's wellbeing. As these conditions face expanding dangers from anthropogenic exercises, contamination, and environmental change, the requirement for viable checking apparatuses becomes fundamental. Inside this biological orchestra, lobsters arise as famous occupants of the ocean as well as sentinel species — cornerstone markers offering significant experiences into the general strength of waterfront environments. This investigation dives into the diverse job of lobsters as sentinels and the significant job they play in checking the wellbeing and flexibility of waterfront conditions.

1. **Cornerstone Species and Environment Wellbeing**
   At the core of each and every environment lies a bunch of cornerstone animal varieties, whose presence and conduct apply lopsided impact on the biological system's design and capability. Lobsters, charming shellfish having a place with the infraorder Astacidea, embody such cornerstone species in beach front environments. Their natural importance is profoundly laced with their differed jobs as hunters, prey, and environment engineers, molding the complex equilibrium of life inside their living spaces.
   Inside the complex food networks of seaside conditions, lobsters go about as dominant hunters, managing the wealth of different species and adding to the general variety and soundness of the environment. As hunters, they assume a significant part in controlling the populaces of different spineless creatures and little fish, impacting the organization of benthic networks and keeping a fragile natural harmony.

2. **Aversion to Natural Changes**
   Lobsters, with their aversion to natural varieties, go about as ecological gauges, reflecting changes in their environmental factors. Their life cycle,

conduct, and physiology are unpredictably connected to natural factors like temperature, saltiness, and water quality. Any changes in these boundaries can have flowing consequences for lobster populaces, making them responsive signs of ecological movements.

Temperature, specifically, arises as a basic variable impacting lobster science. These ectothermic life forms show varieties in development rates, shedding recurrence, and regenerative progress in light of temperature changes. Thusly, observing changes in lobster life history characteristics gives priceless data about the warm states of their living spaces, offering bits of knowledge into more extensive temperature patterns influencing waterfront environments.

3. **Marks of Territory Quality and Contamination**

Lobsters additionally act as sentinels by mirroring the nature of their environments. Their dependence on unambiguous substrates, for example, rough fissure and counterfeit designs, makes them especially receptive to changes in territory quality. Anthropogenic exercises, like seaside advancement, digging, and contamination, can essentially influence lobster natural surroundings, influencing their overflow and dissemination.

In contaminated conditions, lobsters collect impurities in their tissues, giving a bioindicator capability. Weighty metals, pesticides, and different poisons present in beach front waters are consumed by lobsters, mirroring the degree of tainting in their general climate. Checking contamination levels in lobster tissues in this manner turns into a significant device in evaluating the strength of waterfront biological systems and recognizing areas of worry for designated preservation endeavors.

4. **Sickness Elements and Populace Wellbeing**

The soundness of lobster populaces is unpredictably connected to illness elements, making them sentinels for arising wellbeing dangers in beach front biological systems. Lobsters are powerless to different microbes, including microscopic organisms, infections, and parasites, whose predominance and effect can be demonstrative of more extensive biological wellbeing. Changes in illness commonness and power might flag shifts in ecological circumstances, the presentation of obtrusive species, or modifications in have microbe elements inside the biological system.

Observing sickness elements in lobster populaces permits analysts to comprehend the variables impacting illness episodes as well as to survey the general wellbeing and versatility of the beach front biological system. By interpreting the many-sided exchange between natural stressors, have vulnerability, and illness predominance, researchers can acquire a complete comprehension of the multifaceted wellbeing elements inside these touchy biological systems.

5. **Beach front Environment Network**
Lobsters, through their transitory ways of behaving and environment inclinations, go about as couriers of beach front biological system availability. Their developments across various living spaces, going from estuaries to seaward regions, give bits of knowledge into the interconnectedness of assorted biological systems. Cooperative exploration drives that track lobster relocations empower researchers to portray basic environments, grasp the progression of energy and supplements, and distinguish weak regions needing designated protection measures.
Lobsters, in their job as sentinels, overcome any issues between different seaside zones, offering an all encompassing point of view on the wellbeing and versatility of whole environments.
Cooperative endeavors that coordinate information from various districts add to a more nuanced comprehension of waterfront environment elements and help in the improvement of far reaching protection techniques.

6. **Financial Importance and Social Worth**

Past their biological jobs, lobsters hold massive financial importance, especially in seaside networks where lobster fisheries are a foundation of vocations. The soundness of lobster populaces is interlaced with the prosperity of these networks, making them sentinels of environmental wellbeing as well as of financial supportability.

Besides, lobsters bear social importance, frequently filling in as notorious images in the customs and characters of waterfront social orders. Cooperative examination that considers both environmental and socio-social aspects adds to a more all encompassing comprehension of the perplexing connections among people and lobsters. Drawing in with neighborhood networks in checking endeavors guarantees that preservation methodologies line up with the qualities and requirements of individuals who rely upon these marine assets.

1. **Overview of Lobsters as Bioindicators**

In the domain of marine nature, bioindicators assume a pivotal part in unwinding the complexities of ecological wellbeing and quality. Among these bioindicators, lobsters stand apart as alluring and naturally critical organic entities, offering important bits of knowledge into the state of seaside environments. This outline investigates the complex job of lobsters as bioindicators, digging into their physiological reactions, personal conduct standards, and financial ramifications with regards to ecological observing.

1. **The Bioindicator Idea: Evaluating Natural Wellbeing**
   The idea of bioindicators depends on the possibility that specific species show quantifiable reactions to natural changes, making them solid marks of environment wellbeing. In the marine climate, the strength of beach front environments is complicatedly connected to elements like water quality, living space trustworthiness, and the presence of poisons. Lobsters, with their aversion to ecological varieties, act as living checks, mirroring the general wellbeing and nature of their territories.
   As bioindicators, lobsters give a dynamic and constant evaluation of ecological circumstances. Their reactions to changes in temperature, saltiness, contaminations, and illness predominance offer a nuanced comprehension of the complicated cooperations between marine life forms and their environmental elements. Through cooperative examination drives, researchers influence these reactions to check the wellbeing of beach front environments, recognize stressors, and figure out designated protection techniques.

2. **Physiological Reactions: Temperature, pH, and Pollutant Responsiveness**
   Lobsters display perplexing physiological reactions to natural boundaries, making them significant marks of explicit stressors. Temperature, a crucial variable impacting marine life, significantly influences lobster science. Checking the development rates, shedding recurrence, and conceptive outcome of lobster populaces gives experiences into temperature-related pressure and varieties in their natural surroundings.
   Sea fermentation, driven by expanded carbon dioxide retention, is another natural stressor affecting marine life forms. Cooperative examinations including sea life researcher and oceanographers investigate how lobsters answer changes in pH levels. Their aversion to sea fermentation fills in as a mark of more extensive changes in seawater science, giving basic data about the strength of marine biological systems.
   Moreover, lobsters are adroit at amassing pollutants from their current circumstance. Weighty metals, pesticides, and different toxins find their direction into lobster tissues, mirroring the by and large ecological quality. Cooperative examination including physicists, scholars, and natural researchers breaks down these pollutants in lobster tissues to evaluate contamination levels, recognize contamination sources, and guide alleviation endeavors.

3. **Standards of conduct: Marks of Living space Quality and Stressors**
   Lobster conduct fills in as a powerful mark of living space quality and the presence of stressors in waterfront conditions. Their developments, cover inclinations, and taking care of ways of behaving answer changes in natural circumstances, furnishing analysts with significant conduct

measurements for ecological checking.

Cooperative endeavors between marine scientists and behaviorists center around understanding how lobsters explore their territories and answer modifications in substrate quality. Changes in the accessibility of favored cover, substrate sythesis, or natural surroundings construction can impact lobster conduct, flagging changes in environment quality and expected stressors.

Social perceptions additionally add to the ID of anthropogenic effects. Lobsters might change their conduct in light of aggravations like submerged commotion, fishing exercises, or territory modifications. Cooperative examinations including marine environmentalists and fisheries specialists investigate what human exercises mean for lobster conduct, revealing insight into the potential stressors that need alleviation.

4. **Illness Elements: Experiences into Environment Wellbeing**

   Illness elements in lobster populaces offer an extraordinary point of view on the general soundness of beach front biological systems. Cooperative exploration between sea life scientists, veterinarians, and illness environmentalists centers around figuring out the pervasiveness, transmission, and effects of sicknesses in lobster networks.

   Lobsters are powerless to different microbes, including microorganisms, infections, and parasites. Checking infection pervasiveness and concentrating on the cooperations between natural stressors and illness episodes add to a more extensive comprehension of biological system wellbeing. Teammates examine the elements impacting infection elements, evaluate the weakness of lobster populaces, and investigate likely connections between illness designs and more extensive ecological changes.

   By inspecting the complicated interchange between natural stressors, have microbe cooperations, and illness pervasiveness, cooperative exploration drives disentangle the intricate snare of wellbeing elements inside lobster populaces. This comprehensive methodology improves our capacity to anticipate, make due, and relieve sickness influences on seaside biological systems.

5. **Financial Importance: Connecting Natural Wellbeing to Human People group**

   The meaning of lobsters as bioindicators stretches out past biological domains, venturing into the financial texture of beach front networks. Lobster fisheries, a foundation of numerous waterfront economies, depend on solid lobster populaces for supported livelihoods. Cooperative examination including fisheries researchers, financial experts, and social researchers investigates the many-sided associations between lobster wellbeing, fisheries manageability, and the prosperity of human networks.

   Observing the overflow, size conveyance, and conceptive progress of lobster populaces adds to the practical administration of lobster fisheries. Associates work intimately with neighborhood networks to incorporate conventional environmental information and logical bits of knowledge, guaranteeing that protection and the executives systems line up with the qualities and requirements of individuals who rely upon these marine assets.

In addition, lobsters hold social importance in numerous waterfront social orders. Cooperative examinations connect with anthropologists and social specialists to investigate the job of lobsters in nearby customs, craftsmanship, and ceremonies. Understanding the social worth of lobsters improves the inclusivity of protection endeavors, encouraging cooperative methodologies that think about both environmental and human aspects.

6. **Difficulties and Contemplations in Lobster Bioindication**

While lobsters offer significant experiences into beach front environment wellbeing, there are difficulties and contemplations in using them as bioindicators. Cooperative exploration drives should wrestle with the innate fluctuation in lobster populaces, represent local contrasts, and address holes in gauge information. Laying out normalized observing conventions, coordinating different datasets, and cultivating global coordinated efforts upgrade the unwavering quality and equivalence of bioindication endeavors.

Ecological changes, including those determined by environmental change, present extra intricacies. Teammates should explore the synergistic effects of numerous stressors, think about long haul drifts, and expect likely edges past which lobster populaces might confront irreversible decays. This requires interdisciplinary coordinated effort that incorporates environment researchers, biologists, and moderates to foster versatile administration methodologies.

B. Importance of Coastal Ecosystem Health Monitoring

Beach front environments, dynamic and various, act as crucial center points of natural, monetary, and social importance. Be that as it may, the fragile equilibrium of these biological systems is progressively undermined by human exercises, environmental change, and natural debasement. Perceiving the significance of beach front biological systems, checking their wellbeing becomes basic for informed preservation and feasible administration. This investigation digs into the complex significance of beach front biological system wellbeing checking, underscoring its job in supporting biodiversity, supporting vocations, and improving environment flexibility.

1. **Biodiversity Preservation: Saving Biological system Extravagance**
Beach front environments incorporate a rich embroidery of biodiversity, facilitating a large number of animal categories from different scientific

classifications. Mangroves, seagrasses, coral reefs, and estuaries make unpredictable environments that act as nurseries, favorable places, and taking care of regions for various marine and earthbound living beings. The observing of beach front environment wellbeing is fundamental for saving this natural variety, as changes in ecological circumstances can significantly affect the overflow and dissemination of species.

Cooperative endeavors between scientists, sea life scholars, and moderates center around checking key biodiversity pointers, like species lavishness, overflow, and environment quality. Following the soundness of cornerstone species and their communications gives experiences into the general prosperity of the environment. By understanding the elements of beach front biodiversity, scientists and policymakers can configuration designated protection procedures that address explicit dangers and advance the strength of these delicate environments.

2. **Fisheries Maintainability: Supporting Waterfront Jobs**
   Beach front fisheries, frequently entwined with the wellbeing of waterfront environments, give occupations to a large number of individuals around the world. Observing the strength of these environments is essential for supporting fisheries assets and guaranteeing the drawn out prosperity of seaside networks that rely upon them.

   Cooperative exploration including fisheries researchers, oceanographers, and social researchers centers around evaluating fish stocks, understanding relocation designs, and distinguishing potential stressors that might affect fisheries manageability.

   Changes in water quality, territory debasement, and overfishing can have flowing consequences for fish populaces. Seaside environment wellbeing observing works with the early recognition of these stressors, taking into consideration versatile administration methodologies. By incorporating nearby information and logical experiences, partners pursue keeping a fragile harmony between human requirements and the preservation of fisheries assets. Supportable fisheries rehearses, informed by biological system wellbeing observing, add to the strength of both marine environments and the networks that depend on them.

3. **Environment Strength: Relieving the Effects of Environmental Change**
   Seaside biological systems assume a basic part in relieving and adjusting to environmental change. Rising ocean levels, sea fermentation, and outrageous climate occasions present critical dangers to these conditions. Observing seaside environment wellbeing is fundamental for understanding how these biological systems answer environment stressors and for creating techniques to upgrade their flexibility.

   Cooperative exploration drives including environment researchers, biologists, and preservationists plan to survey the weakness of waterfront biological systems to environmental change. Observing changes in ocean level, temperature, and acridity gives important information to foreseeing the effects on marine life and environments. By distinguishing regions in danger, teammates can carry out versatile measures, like living space reclamation, to reinforce the flexibility of seaside biological systems notwithstanding continuous environment challenges.

4. **Water Quality Administration: Protecting Human and Biological system Wellbeing**

The soundness of seaside biological systems is complicatedly connected to water quality, which is fundamental for both environmental equilibrium and human prosperity. Contamination from metropolitan overflow, modern releases, and farming exercises can debase water quality, prompting destructive effects on marine life and beach front environments. Cooperative endeavors between ecological researchers, hydrologists, and policymakers center around observing water quality boundaries to protect the two environments and human wellbeing.

Customary observing of supplement levels, sedimentation rates, and contamination fixations empowers the early recognition of contamination sources. By distinguishing and relieving these sources, teammates make progress toward keeping a good overall arrangement in beach front waters.

The significance of water quality administration reaches out past environmental contemplations, as numerous seaside networks depend on these waters for drinking, entertainment, and social practices.

5. **Disintegration and Living space Misfortune: Saving Beach front Flexibility**

Beach front disintegration and environment misfortune are huge dangers to the solidness and flexibility of seaside biological systems. Regular cycles, intensified by human exercises like urbanization and framework advancement, add to the debasement of coastlines and the deficiency of basic living spaces. Checking the soundness of seaside environments gives essential information to grasping the elements of disintegration and territory misfortune.

Cooperative examination drives including geologists, scientists, and waterfront engineers center around planning changes in coastline morphology, evaluating living space misfortune, and recognizing contributing elements. By understanding the causes and results of disintegration, teammates can carry out measures like seaside reclamation, vegetation the board, and manageable waterfront improvement rehearses. Safeguarding seaside versatility through proactive observing and protection endeavors is fundamental for alleviating the effects of disintegration on the two environments and human networks.

6. Early Admonition Frameworks: Improving Catastrophe Readiness

Beach front regions are powerless against catastrophic events like typhoons, tidal waves, and tempest floods. Checking the soundness of waterfront environments adds to the improvement of early advance notice frameworks that can upgrade calamity readiness and reaction. Cooperative endeavors between meteorologists, biologists, and crisis the executives specialists center around coordinating ecological information into prescient models for catastrophic events.

Changes in seaside environment wellbeing, for example, modifications in mangrove thickness or coral reef structure, can impact the strength of waterfront regions to storm influences. Checking these pointers empowers partners to survey the weakness of beach front environments and, likewise, the networks that possess these locales. Early admonition frameworks, informed by biological system wellbeing observing, give significant lead times to departures, asset allotment, and local area readiness, eventually saving lives and diminishing the effect of catastrophic events.

C. Objectives and Scope of the Book

As we stand at the convergence of natural difficulties and the basic for reasonable works on, understanding and protecting beach front environments have never been more basic. This book intends to dig into the complex universe of beach front environment observing and protection, giving a thorough investigation of its targets, techniques, and the more extensive extent of its suggestions. By winding around together assorted viewpoints, state of the art research, and down to earth experiences, this book tries to engage specialists, policymakers, traditionalists, and the more extensive public with the information and instruments important to defend these essential marine conditions.

1. Characterizing the Targets

1.1. Unwinding the Intricacy of Seaside Biological systems

The essential target of this book is to unwind the intricacy of seaside environments. Waterfront regions, where land meets ocean, are dynamic and many-sided conditions formed by different biological cycles. Grasping the many-sided snare of collaborations among species, living spaces, and ecological variables is critical for powerful preservation. The book means to give a nuanced investigation of the natural elements at play, featuring the interconnectedness of different parts inside seaside biological systems.

1.2. Tending to Arising Natural Difficulties

A key goal is to address arising natural difficulties influencing waterfront biological systems. From environmental change effects on contamination and living space misfortune, seaside conditions face a variety of stressors.

The book tries to dive into these difficulties, presenting top to bottom examinations of their starting points, results, and potential alleviation methodologies. By distinguishing and understanding these difficulties, the book means to add to the advancement of versatile and strong protection draws near.

1.3. Overcoming any barrier among Science and Strategy

Another focal goal is to overcome any barrier between logical exploration and strategy execution. Seaside environment checking creates an abundance of logical information, yet its interpretation into compelling approaches and the board procedures is frequently difficult. This book tries to work with a consistent change from research discoveries to noteworthy strategies. By encouraging interdisciplinary exchange and introducing proof based suggestions, the book looks to engage policymakers in going with informed choices for the preservation and economical utilization of waterfront environments.

1.4. Engaging Neighborhood People group

Enabling nearby networks shapes an essential goal of this book. Seaside people group are in many cases the stewards of these environments, depending on them for occupations and social practices. The book plans to coordinate neighborhood information and points of view, recognizing the significant job of networks in preservation endeavors. By cultivating a feeling of pride and commitment, the book tries to engage nearby networks to become dynamic members in the protection of their waterfront surroundings.

2. Investigating the Extension

2.1. Thorough Inclusion of Seaside Biological system Parts

The extent of the book includes a complete investigation of waterfront environment parts. From mangroves and seagrasses to coral reefs and estuaries, every biological system part assumes a special part in the general strength of waterfront conditions. The book means to give itemized experiences into the environment, biodiversity, and preservation status of these parts, offering a comprehensive comprehension of the variables impacting their elements.

2.2. Coordinating Mechanical Developments in Observing

In the period of mechanical headways, the extension reaches out to the mix of imaginative checking procedures. Remote detecting, submerged advanced mechanics, and information investigation have changed the manner in which we notice and grasp beach front biological systems. The book tries to investigate these advances, underscoring their applications in planning, information assortment, and examination. By displaying the capability of these developments, the book means to motivate further progressions in checking systems.

2.3. Cooperative Contextual investigations and Examples of overcoming adversity

A huge part of the book's degree includes introducing cooperative contextual investigations and examples of overcoming adversity. Beach front biological system protection is in many cases a cooperative exertion including scientists, NGOs, government offices, and nearby networks. The book means to feature fruitful protection drives, representing how cooperation and versatile administration have prompted positive results. By displaying these accounts, the book empowers the replication of successful systems in different beach front settings.

2.4. Moral Contemplations in Protection

Moral contemplations are woven into the texture of the book's degree. As protection endeavors progress, moral inquiries encompassing human instinct collaborations, preservation intercessions, and the evenhanded appropriation of advantages emerge. The book tries to draw in with these moral contemplations, empowering perusers to consider the ethical components of seaside environment preservation. By tending to moral contemplations, the book means to add to the improvement of preservation systems that focus on biological trustworthiness and civil rights.

2.5. Instructive and Effort Drives

The book's extension stretches out to instructive and outreach drives. Information spread is a urgent part of cultivating a culture of protection. The book means to give instructive assets, whether as contextual investigations, infographics, or pragmatic aides, to help learning and mindfulness crusades. By contacting a more extensive crowd, the book tries to impart a feeling of obligation and care for beach front biological systems among understudies, instructors, and the overall population.

3. Techniques and Approaches

3.1. Interdisciplinary Methodologies for All encompassing Getting it

The strategies and approaches embraced in the book are innately interdisciplinary. Waterfront environment checking requires joint effort across disciplines, including nature, oceanography, sociologies, and innovation. The book underlines the significance of interdisciplinary methodologies in accomplishing an all encompassing comprehension of beach front biological systems. By coordinating assorted systems, the book looks to catch the intricacy of these conditions and give nuanced experiences.

3.2. Local area Based Participatory Exploration (CBPR)

Local area based participatory examination (CBPR) is a key methodology implanted in the book's strategies. Perceiving the job of neighborhood networks as basic partners, the book advocates for cooperative exploration models that enable networks. CBPR guarantees that the information and needs of neighborhood networks are vital to the examination cycle.

By integrating CBPR, the book plans to encourage authentic associations, co-make information, and foster setting explicit protection techniques.

3.3. Long haul Checking Projects

Long haul observing projects are vital to the approaches framed in the book. Waterfront environments show dynamic and frequently sluggish paced changes that require supported perception overstretched periods. The book supports the foundation of long haul observing projects, accentuating their part in catching patterns, recognizing abnormalities, and illuminating versatile administration procedures.

By supporting for the congruity of checking endeavors, the book means to add to the advancement of powerful datasets for proof based independent direction.

3.4. Resident Science and Public Commitment

The contribution of residents in logical exploration, known as resident science, is a featured methodology in the book's systems. Connecting with the general population in information assortment, observing, and mindfulness crusades cultivates a feeling of ecological stewardship. The book advocates for resident science drives, giving direction on their execution and exhibiting fruitful models. By empowering public investment, the book tries to intensify the effect of checking endeavors and support an aggregate feeling of obligation for waterfront environments.

4. Future Bearings and Developments

4.1. Expecting Future Difficulties

The book anticipates expecting and tending to future difficulties in waterfront biological system checking and protection. As environmental change speeds up, and human tensions on waterfront regions heighten, the difficulties looked by these biological systems will probably advance. The book means to animate conversations on expected future situations, arising dangers, and creative methodologies to handle forthcoming difficulties. By encouraging a forward-looking viewpoint, the book tries to plan partners for the powerful scene of beach front protection.

4.2. Embracing Innovative Headways

Mechanical headways are a critical concentration later on bearings illustrated fair and square. The fast advancement of innovations like man-made brainpower, satellite imaging, and sensor networks holds enormous potential for altering seaside environment observing. The book intends to investigate these developments, featuring their applications and driving for their joining into standard observing practices. By embracing innovative headways, the book imagines a future where observing is more precise, proficient, and open.

4.3. Mainstreaming Protection Schooling

The future bearings of the book underline mainstreaming protection schooling. As mindfulness turns into an impetus for change, the book imagines a future where protection schooling is incorporated into formal and casual educational plans. By upholding for the consideration of seaside biological system points in instructive projects, the book means to make an age of informed and ecologically cognizant people. This forward-looking methodology underlines the job of training in molding perspectives and ways of behaving towards supportable practices.

4.4. Global Joint effort and Information Trade

Global joint effort and information trade stand apart as key components later on headings illustrated fair and square. Seaside biological systems are interconnected across geological limits, and their protection requires worldwide participation. The book imagines a future where specialists, policymakers, and networks participate in cooperative drives, sharing information, best practices, and illustrations learned. By cultivating global coordinated effort, the book plans to make an organization of help for seaside environments around the world.

CHAPTER 1

Lobster Biology And Behavior

Lobsters, having a place with the family Nephropidae, are captivating scavangers that have caught the interest of researchers, fish devotees, and sea life scientists the same. With their unmistakable appearance and complex ways of behaving, lobsters are central members in marine biological systems as well as assume a huge part in the economy as a significant fish asset. In this investigation, we dig into the complexities of lobster science and conduct, revealing insight into their life structures, life cycle, biological significance, and the captivating social elements that administer their submerged world.

Life systems and Physiology

Exoskeleton and Shedding

One of the characterizing highlights of lobsters is their hard exoskeleton, or shell, which fills in as a defensive external layer. This exoskeleton is fundamentally made out of chitin, an extreme polysaccharide that offers underlying help. In any case, this unbending outside represents a test as lobsters develop. Not at all like warm blooded creatures, lobsters don't develop inside, and their exoskeleton doesn't extend. To oblige development, lobsters go through an interaction called shedding.

Shedding is a pivotal part of lobster science, permitting them to shed their old exoskeleton and structure a bigger one. This cycle is enthusiastically requesting and requires critical assets. Before shedding, lobsters reabsorb calcium carbonate from their old exoskeleton, mellowing it in anticipation of the shed. During the shedding system, lobsters are helpless against predation and frequently look for asylum to limit the dangers related with their briefly delicate bodies.

Tangible Organs

Lobsters have an advanced exhibit of tangible organs, adding to their endurance and route in their marine climate. Their compound eyes, situated on stalks, give a wide field of vision, empowering them to recognize hunters and prey. The eyes are especially delicate to development and changes in light, helping with the identification of likely dangers or open doors.

Notwithstanding their eyes, lobsters have two sets of recieving wires. The principal pair, known as antennules, works fundamentally for olfaction and distinguishing substance prompts in the water. The subsequent pair, radio wires, are associated with contact and taste. These tangible members assume an essential part in correspondence and natural discernment.

Extremities and Motion

Lobsters are furnished with a bunch of strong limbs, each filling a particular need. The main sets of strolling legs, or pereiopods, are adjusted for movement and investigation of their environmental factors. The excess four sets are adjusted for various capabilities, including catching and dealing with food, prepping, and safeguard.

The principal sets of pliers, or chelae, is especially powerful and utilized for catching prey and safeguarding against hunters. The subsequent pair, frequently bigger and more enormous, is adjusted for pounding shells and other hard substances. These transformations are fundamental for the lobster's endurance in its assorted natural specialty.

Life Cycle

Multiplication

Lobsters show a complex conceptive cycle that includes romance, sex, and the arrival of treated eggs. The conceptive cycle starts with romance, where guys take part in presentations of strength and animosity to draw in females. The romance customs include visual and substance signals, with pheromones assuming a significant part in correspondence.

When a female chooses a mate, lovemaking happens, during which the male exchanges sperm to the female. The female then conveys the sperm until she is prepared to deliver her eggs. The treated eggs are conveyed remotely on the female's midsection, safeguarded by a particular design called the "berried" stage. This stage might most recent a while, during which the female gives care and insurance to the creating eggs.

Larval Turn of events

After incubating, lobster hatchlings, known as phyllosoma, go through a progression of formative stages. These stages include shedding, transformation, and changes in morphology. As the hatchlings create, they scatter through the sea flows, benefiting from planktonic life forms. This pelagic stage might keep going for a long time, contingent upon species and ecological circumstances.

After the pelagic stage, the hatchlings settle to the sea depths, going through additional transformation into the adolescent stage. Adolescent lobsters look like smaller than normal adaptations of grown-ups however miss the mark on trademark paws seen in mature people. Over resulting sheds, they foster the famous paws and arrive at sexual development, starting the regenerative cycle once more.

Natural Significance

Cornerstone Species

Lobsters assume a fundamental part in marine biological systems, going about as cornerstone species that impact the overflow and variety of different organic entities. As hunters, lobsters control populaces of more modest spineless creatures, forestalling overgrazing and keeping up with environmental equilibrium. The nonattendance or decline of lobster populaces can prompt flowing impacts on the whole environment, with expected repercussions for financially significant species and the general strength of marine natural surroundings.

Environment Designing

Lobsters are known for their tunneling conduct, making multifaceted homes in the substrate. These tunnels give cover not exclusively to the actual lobsters yet in addition for a horde of other marine living beings. The tunnels act as shelter for little fish, spineless creatures, and adolescent lobsters, offering insurance from hunters and natural stressors. The development and upkeep of tunnels add to the actual design of the natural surroundings, impacting the dispersion and overflow of related species.

Fisheries and Financial Effect

The monetary meaning of lobsters couldn't possibly be more significant. Lobster fisheries are a urgent part of the fish business, giving work and food to beach front networks all over the planet. The ubiquity of lobster as a culinary delicacy has prompted a popularity in worldwide business sectors, driving financial development in districts with vigorous lobster fisheries.

In any case, the maintainability of lobster fisheries is a developing concern. Overfishing, environment annihilation, and environmental change present dangers to lobster populaces and the biological systems they occupy. Protection endeavors and capable administration rehearses are fundamental to guarantee the drawn out reasonability of lobster fisheries and the soundness of marine conditions.

Conduct and Social Elements

Territoriality and Hostility

Lobsters display regional way of behaving, with people marking out and safeguarding explicit region of the sea floor. Regional debates frequently include showcases of animosity, with lobsters utilizing their hooks and non-verbal communication to lay out strength. The size and strength of a singular lobster assume a critical part in deciding its progress in regional challenges.

Regional way of behaving isn't restricted to connections between guys. Female lobsters may likewise show territoriality, particularly during the basic times of romance and mating. These ways of behaving add to the foundation of social orders inside lobster populaces.

Correspondence

Correspondence among lobsters includes a mix of visual, substance, and material signs. Visual presentations, for example, body stances and developments, are vital for conveying strength or accommodation during conflicts. Compound signs, delivered through pee and pheromones, assume a fundamental part in mate choice, romance, and regenerative ways of behaving.

Material correspondence is worked with using radio wires, with lobsters taking part in antennal fencing and shared prepping. Antennal fencing includes people tapping or brushing their radio wires against one another, filling in for the purpose of laying out friendly progressive system and settling debates. Shared preparing is a social way of behaving that builds up friendly bonds inside a gathering.

Social Design

Lobsters display a various leveled social construction in light of size, strength, and predominance. Bigger, all the more influential people will quite often possess the most ideal domains and have more prominent admittance to assets. Social collaborations, for example, strength presentations and regional challenges, assume a significant part in laying out and keeping up with this order.

While lobsters are not exceptionally friendly in the manner that a few well evolved creatures are, they really do display specific helpful ways of behaving. Bunch living gives benefits like expanded insurance from hunters and upgraded scavenging proficiency. In any case, the degree of social collaborations changes among species and is impacted by ecological variables.

Variations to Ecological Difficulties

Osmoregulation

Lobsters are osmoregulators, meaning they effectively manage the salt fixation inside their bodies to keep up with interior equilibrium. In marine conditions, where the outer saltiness can vary, lobsters have developed systems to forestall parchedness and osmotic pressure. Particular gill structures assume a vital part in this cycle, permitting lobsters to discharge overabundance salts while holding fundamental particles.

Thermoregulation

Temperature is a basic element impacting the physiology and conduct of lobsters. As ectothermic creatures, lobsters depend on outside wellsprings of intensity to direct their internal heat level. They are much of the time found in a scope of profundities, choosing natural surroundings that give ideal warm circumstances. Social transformations, like looking for cover or moving to various profundities, permit lobsters to adapt to temperature varieties in their current circumstance.

1.1 Anatomy and Physiology of Lobsters

Lobsters, having a place with the family Nephropidae, are shellfish that show a captivating cluster of physical and physiological transformations. Their many-sided science assumes a urgent part in their endurance, propagation, and connection with their current circumstance. In this complete investigation, we dive into the subtleties of lobster life structures and physiology, looking at their exoskeleton, tangible organs, limbs, regenerative frameworks, and components for osmoregulation and thermoregulation.

Exoskeleton and Shedding

Primary Structure

A characterizing component of lobsters is their exoskeleton, an outside covering that offers help, security, and a boundary against ecological difficulties. Made essentially out of chitin, an extreme polysaccharide, the exoskeleton is liable for the unbending external shell that describes lobsters and different scavangers.

Chitin gives strength and adaptability, permitting lobsters to keep up with their shape and safeguard their inside organs. The exoskeleton is coordinated into unmistakable districts, with explained joints that work with development. The unbending nature of the exoskeleton is a consequence of the mineralization of chitin with calcium carbonate, giving extra strength and sturdiness.

Shedding Cycle

One of the most exceptional parts of lobster science is the shedding system, which permits these shellfish to develop and adjust to changing natural circumstances. Not at all like vertebrates, lobsters don't have inside skeletons, and their exoskeleton doesn't develop with them. In this manner, shedding is an imperative component for development.

The shedding system, or ecdysis, includes the shedding of the old exoskeleton and the development of a bigger one. Preceding shedding, lobsters start a progression of physiological changes. They reabsorb calcium carbonate from the current exoskeleton, relaxing it and planning for the shed. The retention of minerals is an asset escalated cycle, and lobsters frequently eat a lot of calcium-rich food in anticipation of shedding.

During shedding, lobsters are profoundly powerless against predation and ecological pressure. They look for haven to limit gambles, and the shedding system itself is a painstakingly coordinated succession of occasions. The lobster secretes chemicals that digest the internal layers of the exoskeleton, permitting it to rise up out of the old shell. The new exoskeleton, at first delicate and flexible, step by step solidifies and calcifies throughout the next days.

Shedding is a huge energy use for lobsters, and the recurrence of shedding shifts with age and natural variables. Youthful lobsters shed all the more as often as possible as they experience quick development, while more seasoned people might shed less habitually.

Tactile Organs

Compound Eyes

Lobsters are furnished with compound eyes, a typical component among arthropods. Their eyes are arranged on stalks, taking into consideration a wide field of vision. Each eye comprises of various ommatidia, individual visual units that by and large structure the compound eye. The plan of ommatidia empowers lobsters to recognize movement and changes in light force, furnishing them with an uplifted consciousness of their environmental elements.

According to lobsters are especially delicate to energized light, supporting route and direction. This responsiveness is vital for recognizing hunters and prey and assumes a part in the complex visual presentations saw during romance and other social cooperations.

Recieving wires and Antennules

Lobsters have two sets of recieving wires — long, slim members that assume fundamental parts in tactile discernment. The main pair, known as antennules, are more modest and arranged before the bigger radio wires. Antennules capability essentially in olfaction, permitting lobsters to identify substance prompts in the water.

The subsequent pair, the recieving wires, are bigger and more strong. They serve various capabilities, including contact, taste, and the recognition of mechanical upgrades. Lobsters utilize their recieving wires to investigate their current circumstance, find food, and participate in material correspondence with different lobsters.

Extremities and Headway

Pereiopods

Lobsters have ten strolling legs, aggregately alluded to as pereiopods, organized in five sets. The initial three sets are prepared for strolling and are usually utilized for investigating the sea floor and catching prey.

The design of these strolling legs incorporates sections with joints, taking into consideration a large number of developments.

The fourth and fifth sets of pereiopods are changed into chelae, or paws, which assume specific parts in taking care of, safeguard, and social communications. The principal sets of paws is generally bigger and more grounded, adjusted for squashing and cutting. The subsequent pair might be more able, with better ways to deal with food and different items.

Chelae

The chelae, or hooks, are one of the most unmistakable highlights of lobsters. They are strong and flexible extremities that serve different capabilities. The main pair, frequently alluded to as the smasher paw, is adjusted for pounding hard substances, like the shells of mollusks and scavangers. The subsequent pair, known as the shaper paw, is furnished with better, more pointed tips, considering accuracy in taking care of and cutting.

The chelae are fundamental for taking care of, as lobsters are basically scroungers and hunters. They utilize their hooks to catch and control prey, as well as to fall to pieces shells to get to the delicate tissue inside. The chelae likewise assume a significant part in regional debates and romance customs, where lobsters use them to state strength or draw in mates.

Life Cycle

Proliferation

The conceptive course of lobsters is a perplexing and multifaceted series of ways of behaving and physiological changes. Propagation is ordinarily started by visual and synthetic signs, with romance customs filling in as the antecedent to fornication.

Romance ways of behaving include showcases of predominance, hostility, and visual signs to draw in possible mates. Male lobsters frequently participate in battle, utilizing their paws and non-verbal communication to lay out predominance and win the blessing of females. Pheromones assume an essential part in compound correspondence, helping with the ID of reasonable mates.

When romance is effective, sex happens, during which the male exchanges sperm to the female. Female lobsters convey the sperm until they are prepared to deliver their eggs. The female then enters the berried stage, portrayed by the presence of a mass of treated eggs joined to her midsection. During this stage, which might most recent a while, the female gives care and security to the creating eggs.

Larval Turn of events

After bring forth, lobster hatchlings, known as phyllosoma, enter a pelagic stage where they float with sea flows. This stage is described by a progression of sheds and transformative changes. The hatchlings go through a few progressive phases, each undeniable by unmistakable morphological elements.

As phyllosoma hatchlings, lobsters are channel feeders, drinking planktonic life forms present in the water section. This pelagic stage is critical for the dispersal of hatchlings, permitting them to colonize new regions and adding to quality stream inside lobster populaces.

After the pelagic stage, the hatchlings go through transformation, progressing into the adolescent stage. Adolescent lobsters settle to the sea floor, where they proceed to develop and create. Over ensuing sheds, they obtain the trademark elements of grown-up lobsters, including the improvement of paws.

Environmental Significance

Cornerstone Species

Lobsters are perceived as cornerstone species in marine biological systems, applying huge impact on the overflow and circulation of different species. As hunters, lobsters assume a pivotal part in controlling the populaces of more modest spineless creatures. This predation keeps up with biological equilibrium by forestalling overgrazing and guaranteeing the wellbeing of marine territories.

The expulsion or decline of lobster populaces can prompt flowing impacts inside environments. Without the directing impact of lobsters, certain invertebrate populaces might multiply, adversely influencing different species and modifying the construction of marine networks.

Territory Designing

The tunneling conduct of lobsters adds to territory designing, forming the actual construction of the sea depths. Lobsters make unpredictable tunnels in the substrate, giving sanctuary to themselves and various other marine life forms. These tunnels act as significant natural surroundings for little fish, spineless creatures, and adolescent lobsters, offering insurance from hunters and ecological stressors.

The development and upkeep of tunnels likewise add to residue turnover, impacting supplement cycling and the structure of benthic networks. The presence of lobster tunnels improves the general biodiversity and efficiency of marine territories.

Fisheries and Financial Effect

Lobsters hold colossal monetary significance as an important fish asset. Lobster fisheries contribute fundamentally to the worldwide fish industry, giving work, food, and financial open doors for beach front networks.

The prominence of lobster as a culinary delicacy has prompted a popularity in global business sectors, driving financial development in locales with flourishing lobster fisheries.

In any case, the maintainability of lobster fisheries is a developing concern. Overfishing, environment annihilation, and environmental change present dangers to lobster populaces and the biological systems they occupy. Capable administration rehearses, preservation endeavors, and the foundation of marine safeguarded regions are fundamental to guarantee the drawn out feasibility of lobster fisheries.

Conduct and Social Elements

Territoriality and Hostility

Lobsters display regional way of behaving, with people marking out and safeguarding explicit region of the sea depths. Regional debates are normal and frequently include showcases of hostility, with lobsters utilizing their paws and non-verbal communication to lay out predominance.

Male lobsters, specifically, take part in forceful ways of behaving during romance, vieing for the consideration of females. Battle includes wrestling with hooks and actual posing, with the victor accessing regenerative open doors. Territoriality reaches out past romance, impacting the conveyance of people inside a populace.

Female lobsters may likewise show regional way of behaving, particularly during the berried stage while safeguarding eggs. Regional questions among females can happen, and admittance to reasonable settling locales might turn into a disputed matter.

Correspondence

Correspondence among lobsters includes a mix of visual, synthetic, and material signs. Visual presentations, for example, body stances and developments, assume a urgent part in conveying predominance or accommodation during conflicts. Lobsters utilize their compound eyes to identify these visual signs, taking into consideration quick and nuanced correspondence.

Compound signs, delivered through pee and pheromones, assume an imperative part in mate choice, romance, and conceptive ways of behaving. Pheromones produced by females in the berried stage draw in guys and act as marks of regenerative status. Male lobsters discharge pee containing substance prompts that pass on data about their size, wellbeing, and strength.

Material correspondence is worked with using radio wires. Lobsters participate in antennal fencing, a way of behaving where people tap or brush their recieving wires against one another. Antennal fencing fills in for of laying out friendly ordered progression, settling debates, and passing on data about conceptive status.

Shared preparing is one more type of material correspondence saw among lobsters. This conduct includes people utilizing their strolling legs and chelae to clean and prepare one another. Shared preparing builds up friendly bonds inside a gathering and adds to the support of a durable social construction.

Social Construction

Lobsters display a progressive social design in light of size, strength, and predominance. Bigger, all the more influential people will generally possess the most good regions and have more prominent admittance to assets. Social connections, for example, strength showcases and regional challenges, assume a significant part in laying out and keeping up with this pecking order.

While lobsters are not exceptionally friendly in the manner that a few vertebrates are, they really do display specific helpful ways of behaving. Bunch living gives benefits like expanded assurance from hunters and upgraded scrounging productivity. Lobsters might assemble in protected regions, framing free conglomerations that adjustment of creation over the long haul.

The social construction of lobster populaces can be dynamic, with people moving among gatherings and domains in view of changes in size, regenerative status, or ecological circumstances. Social elements assume a critical part in the general working of lobster populaces and add to the strength of these life forms in their marine surroundings.

Variations to Ecological Difficulties

Osmoregulation

Osmoregulation is the cycle by which lobsters effectively manage the salt fixation inside their bodies to keep up with inner equilibrium. In marine conditions, where the outside saltiness can fluctuate, lobsters have advanced components to forestall lack of hydration and osmotic pressure.

The gills of lobsters assume a vital part in osmoregulation. Specific designs inside the gills effectively transport particles, permitting lobsters to discharge abundance salts while holding fundamental particles. This transformation empowers lobsters to keep up with osmotic equilibrium in different saltiness conditions, from the untamed sea to estuarine conditions.

Lobsters are likewise fit for changing their osmoregulatory systems in light of changes in saltiness. This adaptability permits them to adjust to various natural surroundings and endure changes in ecological circumstances.

Thermoregulation

Temperature is a basic element impacting the physiology and conduct of lobsters. As ectothermic life forms, lobsters depend on outside wellsprings of intensity to direct their internal heat level. They are in many cases found in a scope of profundities, choosing environments that give ideal warm circumstances.

Social transformations assume a pivotal part in thermoregulation. Lobsters might look for cover in cleft or tunnels to keep away from outrageous temperatures or predation. They may likewise move to various profundities inside the water segment, where temperature slopes exist. Vertical relocation permits lobsters to get to hotter or cooler waters, contingent upon their physiological requirements.

Notwithstanding social transformations, physiological components add to thermoregulation. The action level of lobsters is affected by temperature, with varieties in metabolic rates saw at various warm circumstances. As temperature influences different physiological cycles, lobsters show an ability to adjust to changes in their current circumstance.

1.2 Unique Features that Make Lobsters Effective Sentinels

Lobsters, with their complicated science and complex ways of behaving, act as something other than culinary pleasures. These shellfish assume a critical part as sentinels in marine biological systems, going about as signs of natural wellbeing and giving significant experiences into the condition of the seas. In this investigation, we dive into the exceptional highlights that make lobsters viable sentinels, looking at their aversion to natural changes, jobs as cornerstone species, and commitments to logical examination and protection endeavors.

1. **Aversion to Ecological Changes**

   Lobsters show a noteworthy aversion to natural changes, making them viable signs of movements in maritime circumstances. Their dependence on unambiguous temperature ranges, saltiness levels, and territory highlights renders them exceptionally powerless to modifications in their environmental elements. Checking lobster populaces can accordingly uncover significant data about more extensive changes in the marine climate.

Thermosensitivity

One of the key variables adding to the responsiveness of lobsters is their thermosensitivity. These shellfish are ectothermic, meaning their inside internal heat level is affected by the outside climate. In that capacity, they are exceptionally sensitive to temperature vacillations, and modifications past their ideal reach can affect their digestion, development, and conduct.

Warming sea temperatures, a result of environmental change, straightforwardly influence the physiology of lobsters. Changes in water temperature can impact shedding cycles, regenerative examples, and generally speaking metabolic rates. Concentrating on these impacts gives researchers important information on the effect of environmental change on marine life forms.

Osmoregulation Elements

Lobsters are likewise especially delicate to changes in saltiness. Osmoregulation, the interaction by which they direct salt fixation inside their bodies, is finely tuned to the particular saltiness levels of their natural surroundings. An awkwardness in saltiness can prompt osmotic pressure, influencing the lobsters' capacity to keep up with water balance and disturbing their physiological capabilities.

Checking varieties in saltiness resilience and osmoregulatory reactions in lobster populaces can give bits of knowledge into the wellbeing of estuarine conditions and the effects of human exercises, for example, modern overflow or changes in freshwater input, on waterfront biological systems.

Natural surroundings Inclinations

Lobsters are exceptionally specific in their selection of natural surroundings. Their inclination for explicit substrate types and the accessibility of reasonable safe houses impact their circulation. Natural modifications, like environment debasement or changes in substrate arrangement, can bring about shifts in lobster populaces.

Noticing these movements can act as an early advance notice framework, making specialists aware of potential issues influencing the general soundness of marine environments. Lobsters, in this sense, go about as natural sentinels, flagging changes in their living space that might include more extensive ramifications for different species inside the biological system.

2. **Cornerstone Species Status**

Lobsters stand firm on an essential footing as cornerstone species inside marine biological systems. Cornerstone species apply unbalanced impact on their current circumstance, and changes in their populaces can have flowing impacts all through the biological system. The job of lobsters as cornerstone species upgrades their viability as sentinels of ecological wellbeing.

Ruthless Control

As hunters, lobsters assume a fundamental part in controlling the populaces of more modest spineless creatures. By going after life forms, for example, ocean imps and crabs, lobsters forestall overgrazing and keep up with the equilibrium of the environment.

At the point when lobster populaces decline because of variables like overfishing or territory corruption, the unrestrained multiplication of specific spineless creatures can happen, prompting the debasement of natural surroundings, for example, kelp woodlands.

Checking lobster populaces gives experiences into the condition of ruthless control inside a biological system. A decrease in lobster numbers might show uneven characters that could have broad results, impacting the overflow and variety of different species inside the local area.

Territory Designing

The tunneling conduct of lobsters adds to the actual construction of marine territories. Lobsters make perplexing tunnels in the substrate, giving haven to themselves and various other marine life forms. These tunnels act as significant territories for little fish, spineless creatures, and adolescent lobsters, offering security from hunters and natural stressors.

Changes in the commonness of lobster tunnels can demonstrate adjustments in environment quality and accessibility. Concentrating on the appropriation of tunnels can give significant data about the soundness of benthic environments and the effect of human exercises on these indispensable territories.

Biodiversity and Trophic Fountains

The presence or nonattendance of lobsters can impact the general biodiversity of marine environments. Their savage job manages the overflow of specific species, forestalling the predominance of a couple and advancing a more different local area. The gradually expanding influences of these trophic communications can shape the construction of whole biological systems.

Changes in lobster populaces can set off trophic fountains, where changes in one trophic level impact ensuing levels in the food web. Understanding these fountains is fundamental for appreciating the many-sided connections inside marine environments. Lobsters, going about as cornerstone species, assist scientists with following these elements and evaluate the general wellbeing and versatility of environments.

3. **Commitments to Logical Exploration**

Lobsters contribute essentially to logical examination, filling in as important subjects for concentrates on in different fields. Their novel elements make them ideal possibility for examinations concerning physiological cycles, conduct, and the effects of ecological stressors.

Shedding as a Development Marker

The shedding system of lobsters, a vital part of their science, offers experiences into development rates and ecological circumstances. By analyzing the recurrence and timing of sheds, scientists can survey the effect of elements like temperature, food accessibility, and territory quality on lobster populaces.

Shedding likewise gives a window into the conceptive strength of lobster populaces. Changes in the shedding cycle can be characteristic of stressors, illnesses, or disturbances in the conceptive cycle. By observing shedding designs, researchers gain a more profound comprehension of the variables impacting lobster populaces and their versatility to natural changes.

Conduct Reactions to Stressors

Lobsters show complex ways of behaving that can be firmly seen to check their reactions to natural stressors. Changes in taking care of examples, development, and conceptive ways of behaving can be characteristic of aggravations in their environment. Concentrating on these social reactions permits researchers to recognize stressors, survey their effect, and foster methodologies for preservation and the executives.

Bioindicators of Foreign substance Openness

Lobsters likewise act as bioindicators of impurity openness in marine conditions. Their capacity to aggregate poisons, for example, weighty metals and natural mixtures, in their tissues makes them important signs of water quality. Checking pollutant levels in lobster populaces gives essential information on the strength of the environment and expected dangers to human wellbeing through fish utilization.

4. **Preservation Endeavors and The executives Systems**

The exceptional highlights of lobsters put forth them integral to protection attempts and the advancement of reasonable administration systems. By figuring out their science, conduct, and reactions to natural changes, analysts and policymakers can execute measures to guarantee the drawn out wellbeing and versatility of lobster populaces.

Fishery The board

Lobster fisheries are indispensable for the overwhelming majority waterfront networks, giving financial open doors and supporting jobs. In any case, the maintainability of these fisheries is dependent upon powerful administration rehearses. Understanding the existence cycle, conceptive science, and conduct of lobsters empowers policymakers to carry out measures, for example, size limits, occasional terminations, and marine safeguarded regions to shield populaces and forestall overfishing.

Territory Security

Given the significance of lobster tunnels as territories for different marine living beings, environment insurance is a basic part of preservation endeavors. Distinguishing key regions for insurance in view of lobster living space necessities adds to the conservation of biodiversity and the general soundness of marine biological systems.

Environmental Change Transformation

As sentinels of environmental change, lobsters give urgent data about the effects of increasing temperatures and changing sea conditions. Protection endeavors should incorporate techniques to address environment related difficulties, like territory misfortune, modified conceptive examples, and changes in dissemination. Versatile administration approaches can assist with relieving the impacts of environmental change on lobster populaces.

1.3 Behavioral Patterns and Interactions in Coastal Environments

Seaside conditions are dynamic and rich biological systems where a bunch of standards of conduct and cooperations among marine creatures shape the perplexing embroidery of life. From the clamoring action of searching and taking care of to the complexities of romance ceremonies and regional questions, the social elements in waterfront biological systems offer a captivating look into the perplexing connections that oversee marine life. In this investigation, we dig into the standards of conduct and cooperations of different species in seaside conditions, featuring the vital job they play in the working and versatility of these biological systems.

Scrounging and Taking care of Procedures

Scrounging and taking care of ways of behaving are fundamental to the endurance of marine organic entities in beach front conditions. The accessibility of food assets, going from planktonic creatures to bigger prey, impacts the procedures utilized by various species.

Channel Taking care of and Suspension Taking care of

In seaside waters, channel feeders flourish with tiny organic entities suspended in the water section. Bivalves, for example, mussels and shellfish, utilize particular designs to channel tiny fish and natural particles from the water. These channel taking care of life forms add to the refinement of beach front waters and partake in supplement cycling.

Essentially, a few marine spineless creatures, similar to specific types of wipes and tunicates, participate in suspension taking care of. They extricate supplements from water by siphoning it through particular designs and sifting through particles. These ways of behaving support the life forms themselves as well as impact the general water quality in seaside environments.

Ruthless Ways of behaving

Predation is an unavoidable part of waterfront conditions, with a different cluster of hunters focusing on different prey things. Seaside waters abound with savage fish, cephalopods, and scavangers took part in pursuits and ambushes. The hunting techniques utilized by these life forms are essentially as different as the beach front territories they occupy.

A few hunters, like beach front sharks, use secrecy and explosions of speed to get prey. Others, similar to loner crabs, rummage for flesh along the coastlines. The exchange among hunters and prey shapes populace elements and impacts the appropriation of species in waterfront environments.

Regenerative Ways of behaving and Romance Ceremonies

Seaside conditions act as pivotal favorable places for the majority marine species, and regenerative ways of behaving and romance ceremonies are indispensable parts of the existence cycle.

Settling and Generating Ways of behaving

Various fish species use waterfront conditions for settling and generating. During the reproducing season, male fish might make homes on the substrate, frequently in shallow waters. They participate in romance showcases to draw in females, and the fruitful matching outcomes in the statement of eggs in the homes.

A notable model is the way of behaving of certain types of salmon. These fish embrace noteworthy excursions from the vast sea to waterfront waterways to produce. The complexities of their upstream relocation, choice of settling destinations, and romance showcases are fundamental parts of the seaside biological system's regenerative elements.

Regional Shows and Mate Determination

In seaside conditions, regional way of behaving and mate choice are frequently seen among different species. Shorebirds, for example, take part in intricate romance presentations and vocalizations to draw in mates and lay out domains along the shoreline. Matches protect their settling destinations against gatecrashers, showing the significance of spatial association in waterfront rearing regions.

Ocean turtles, another model, display explicit ways of behaving during the settling system. Female turtles return to explicit sea shores to lay their eggs, participating in fastidious settling customs. The determination of settling destinations and the resulting development of hatchlings are basic parts of the regenerative nature of ocean turtles in beach front conditions.

Social Cooperations and Collective vibes

Social cooperations and collective vibes assume a critical part in the existences of numerous waterfront life forms. From the planned developments of tutoring fish to the agreeable ways of behaving of marine warm blooded animals, these social designs upgrade endurance and add to the environmental equilibrium of seaside biological systems.

Tutoring and Shoaling

Tutoring and shoaling ways of behaving are common among fish species in seaside waters. These aggregate ways of behaving give benefits like expanded security from hunters, upgraded scrounging effectiveness, and further developed route.

Fish schools, where people swim in an organized way, act as both a cautious system and a method for finding prey. Sandbars, portrayed by approximately accumulated gatherings, are many times seen in seaside regions where fish assemble for taking care of or propagation. The synchronicity of these ways of behaving is a hypnotizing sight and a demonstration of the versatility of marine life forms in unique seaside conditions.

Helpful Taking care of and Hunting

Helpful taking care of and hunting ways of behaving are seen in different marine species along the coast. Seaside dolphins, for instance, participate in helpful hunting to corral and catch schools of fish. The coordinated effort among people takes into account the effective use of assets and the fruitful catch of prey.

Likewise, some bird species, like pelicans and gulls, show helpful taking care of ways of behaving. They coordinate their developments to trap and focus schools of fish, making it more straightforward for them to catch their prey. These agreeable methodologies are fundamental for enhancing taking care of chances in waterfront environments.

Territoriality and Forceful Associations

Territoriality and forceful communications are normal highlights in beach front conditions, where restricted assets and appropriate living spaces can prompt rivalry among people.

Regional Showcases and Guard

Numerous seaside creatures, from crabs to shorebirds, participate in regional showcases to lay out and shield their domains. These presentations frequently include visual signs, vocalizations, or actual showdowns to hinder likely interlopers.

Recluse crabs, for example, may participate in forceful communications over the inhabitance of empty shells, a basic asset for their security. In beach front bird states, people protect settling destinations against rivals, exhibiting elaborate shows and participating in forceful ways of behaving to keep up with elite admittance to rearing regions.

Contest for Assets

Contest for assets, for example, settling locales, food, and reproducing regions, is a main thrust behind forceful cooperations in waterfront biological systems. Seabird provinces along waterfront precipices might observer extraordinary rivalry for prime settling areas, prompting conflicts and shows of strength.

Likewise, in intertidal zones, where assets are restricted, crabs and different shellfish might contend forcefully for admittance to concealing spots, food, and mates. These serious collaborations impact populace elements and asset usage in beach front conditions.

Variations to Anthropogenic Impacts

Beach front conditions face expanding anthropogenic tensions, going from contamination to natural surroundings annihilation. The social variations of marine creatures to these difficulties give significant experiences into their flexibility and ability to coincide with human exercises.

Social Reactions to Contamination

Marine creatures in seaside conditions exhibit different conduct reactions to contamination. A few animal categories show evasion ways of behaving, creating some distance from regions with high contamination fixations. Others might modify their taking care of techniques or regenerative ways of behaving in light of the presence of impurities.

Fish, for instance, may change their searching areas or taking care of profundities in light of contamination. Also, shellfish might change their tunneling ways of behaving to keep away from defiled residue. Concentrating on these social reactions supports evaluating the effect of contamination on beach front biological systems and the adequacy of preservation measures.

Changed Relocation and Development Examples

Anthropogenic impacts, like beach front turn of events and transportation exercises, can upset the relocation and development examples of marine life forms. A few animal varieties might modify their courses or timing of relocation in light of expanded human exercises.

Marine warm blooded animals, including whales and dolphins, may display changes in their dispersion and development examples to keep away from regions with weighty sea traffic. Understanding these variations is pivotal for executing preservation gauges and alleviating the effect of human exercises on seaside species.

CHAPTER 2

Coastal Ecosystems And Environmental Challenges

Waterfront biological systems are dynamic and various conditions where land and ocean unite, leading to rich biodiversity and giving a huge number of natural administrations. Notwithstanding, these significant biological systems are confronting a variety of natural difficulties that undermine their wellbeing and usefulness. From territory debasement to contamination and environmental change, the fragile equilibrium of waterfront biological systems is in danger. In this investigation, we dive into the complexities of seaside biological systems, their significance, and the squeezing ecological difficulties they defy.

The Significance of Seaside Environments

Seaside environments incorporate a large number of living spaces, including mangroves, estuaries, intertidal zones, and coral reefs. These regions are portrayed by their nearness to the point of interaction of land and ocean, establishing a one of a kind and dynamic climate that upholds a horde of living things. The meaning of waterfront environments stretches out past their stylish worth, assuming an essential part in natural cycles, biodiversity protection, and the prosperity of human networks.

Biodiversity Areas of interest

Beach front biological systems are perceived as biodiversity areas of interest, holding onto a lopsidedly big number of species in contrast with their topographical size. Mangroves, for instance, give significant nursery living spaces to various fish species, supporting the beginning phases of their life cycles. Coral reefs, frequently alluded to as the "rainforests of the ocean," have an inconceivable variety of marine life, including different fish, spineless creatures, and coral species.

This abundance of biodiversity adds to the strength of seaside biological systems, upgrading their ability to adjust to natural changes. The interconnectedness of species inside these biological systems makes unpredictable food networks and natural connections that control supplement cycling, populace elements, and generally speaking environment wellbeing.

Financial and Cultural Advantages

Beach front biological systems give a wide cluster of environment benefits that are fundamental for human prosperity and financial exercises. Fisheries, upheld by the efficiency of beach front waters, are a significant wellspring of food and vocations for waterfront networks around the world. Numerous industrially significant fish species depend on seaside environments for producing, nursery grounds, and taking care of.

Moreover, waterfront biological systems go about as regular supports against tempests and disintegration. Mangroves and salt bogs, with their thick underground roots, assist with disseminating wave energy and lessen the effect of tempest floods. This regular security is basic for seaside networks, shielding framework and decreasing the dangers related with outrageous climate occasions.

The travel industry, another critical financial driver, depends intensely on the allure of seaside conditions. Perfect sea shores, dynamic coral reefs, and various marine life draw in large number of sightseers every year, adding to nearby economies and producing income for protection drives.

Ecological Difficulties Confronting Seaside Biological systems

Notwithstanding their natural and monetary significance, waterfront biological systems are confronting a variety of ecological difficulties that undermine their trustworthiness and versatility. These difficulties emerge from both normal cycles and anthropogenic exercises, aggregately presenting dangers to the wellbeing and maintainability of waterfront conditions.

Natural surroundings Debasement and Misfortune

Living space corruption and misfortune are among the chief difficulties facing seaside environments. Urbanization, rural extension, and foundation advancement frequently bring about the change of normal environments into human-overwhelmed scenes. Mangrove timberlands, estuarine wetlands, and waterfront hills are especially defenseless against environment misfortune because of these exercises.

The evacuation of mangrove woods for hydroponics lakes, for instance, prompts the deficiency of biodiversity as well as lessens the environment administrations given by mangroves, like tempest insurance and water filtration. The depleting of wetlands for farming purposes upsets fundamental reproducing and taking care of reason for various bird species and other amphibian living beings.

Waterfront urbanization, energized by populace development and financial turn of events, frequently prompts the recovery of beach front regions for foundation projects. This adjustment of normal shorelines lessens natural surroundings accessibility as well as upsets the complex equilibrium of biological systems and can intensify the effects of environmental change.

Contamination: Land-Based and Marine

Contamination represents an unavoidable danger to waterfront environments, appearing in different structures, for example, supplement spillover, sedimentation, oil slicks, and plastic contamination. Land-based wellsprings of contamination, including agrarian spillover and untreated sewage, present overabundance supplements like nitrogen and phosphorus into waterfront waters.

Exorbitant supplement data sources can prompt eutrophication, a peculiarity where algal sprouts multiply, draining oxygen levels in the water and causing "no man's lands" where marine life can't make due. This has significant ramifications for fish and invertebrate populaces, disturbing the equilibrium of beach front biological systems.

Oil slicks, whether from modern exercises, delivering mishaps, or normal leaks, can horrendous affect seaside biological systems. The poisonousness of oil mixtures can hurt marine life at different trophic levels, from phytoplankton to fish and seabirds. Long haul results remember the industriousness of oil deposits for silt and the sluggish recuperation of impacted environments.

Plastic contamination is another major problem influencing waterfront conditions. Plastics, particularly single-use things, collect in seaside waters, representing a danger to marine life through ingestion and ensnarement. Microplastics, coming about because of the breakdown of bigger plastic things, further pervade marine biological systems, influencing creatures at the minuscule level.

Overfishing and Impractical Gathering

Overfishing and impractical gathering rehearses present critical dangers to the biodiversity and environmental equilibrium of waterfront biological systems. Numerous industrially significant fish species depend on seaside environments for producing and nursery grounds. Overexploitation of these areas can prompt decreases in fish populaces, influencing the designated species as well as the more extensive marine food web.

The utilization of disastrous fishing rehearses, for example, impact fishing and base fishing, can make actual harm ocean bottom environments, including coral reefs and seagrass beds. These territories act as fundamental reproducing and taking care of justification for different marine species. Disastrous fishing rehearses drain target species as well as result in blow-back to non-designated species and natural surroundings.

Environmental Change Effects: Climbing Temperatures and Ocean Level Ascent

Environmental change is intensifying the difficulties looked by beach front biological systems, with climbing temperatures and ocean level ascent being unmistakable effects. Raised ocean surface temperatures can prompt coral blanching, a peculiarity where cooperative green growth residing inside coral tissues are ousted, making the corals lose their dynamic tones and expanding their weakness to infections.

Ocean level ascent represents an immediate danger to low-lying seaside territories, including mangroves, salt bogs, and sandy sea shores. As ocean levels rise, these living spaces might become lowered, prompting territory misfortune and the uprooting of related species. Furthermore, ocean level ascent can strengthen the effects of tempest floods, compounding seaside disintegration and undermining human settlements.

Sea Fermentation

Sea fermentation, coming about because of the ingestion of overabundance carbon dioxide via seawater, is a worldwide test with especially articulated influences on beach front environments. The fermentation of seawater can adversely influence marine living beings with calcium carbonate skeletons or shells, like corals, mollusks, and a few planktonic animal types.

Corals, fundamental parts of coral reefs, face decreased calcification rates, thwarting their capacity to construct and keep up with their calcium carbonate structures. Also, shell-shaping living beings, including clams and specific sorts of microscopic fish, may encounter hardships in shell development, affecting their endurance and conceptive achievement.

Protection and Relief Techniques for Seaside Environments

Tending to the ecological difficulties confronting seaside environments requires far reaching and incorporated preservation and relief procedures. These techniques envelop living space security, supportable asset the board, contamination avoidance, and environmental change variation.

Marine Safeguarded Regions (MPAs) and Natural surroundings Rebuilding

Laying out Marine Safeguarded Regions (MPAs) is a critical methodology for defending waterfront environments. MPAs can act as shelters for marine life, permitting populaces to recuperate and territories to recover. Safeguarding basic territories, for example, mangroves, seagrass beds, and coral reefs, inside these assigned regions is fundamental for keeping up with biodiversity and biological system flexibility.

Environment reclamation drives assume a pivotal part in switching the effects of living space debasement. Endeavors to replant mangroves, reestablish seagrass knolls, and restore coral reefs add to the recuperation of seaside environments. These drives frequently include coordinated effort between neighborhood networks, state run administrations, and protection associations.

Economical Fisheries The executives

Carrying out reasonable fisheries the board rehearses is fundamental for keeping up with the strength of seaside biological systems and guaranteeing the drawn out practicality of fish populaces. This incorporates setting and authorizing fishing portions, executing gear limitations to limit territory harm, and advancing particular fishing rehearses that lessen bycatch.

Connecting with nearby networks in feasible fisheries the board is basic for the progress of protection endeavors. Local area based drives, like co-administration frameworks, enable nearby fishers to effectively partake in dynamic cycles, cultivating a feeling of pride and obligation regarding the prosperity of beach front biological systems.

Contamination Avoidance and Cleanup

Endeavors to forestall and alleviate contamination in waterfront conditions require multi-layered approaches. Executing appropriate waste administration works on, diminishing the utilization of single-use plastics, and putting resources into wastewater treatment offices are fundamental parts of contamination anticipation.

Local area commitment and training assume a vital part in bringing issues to light about the effects of contamination and advancing capable way of behaving. Seaside cleanup drives, including neighborhood networks and volunteers, add to the expulsion of marine trash and plastic waste from beach front regions.

Environmental Change Transformation and Relief

Tending to the effects of environmental change on seaside biological systems requires both transformation and relief techniques. Variation measures incorporate the insurance and rebuilding of beach front territories that go about as normal cushions against storm floods and disintegration. Waterfront zone arranging that considers projected ocean level ascent is significant for practical turn of events.

Moderating environmental change requires worldwide endeavors to decrease ozone harming substance discharges. Progressing to environmentally friendly power sources, upgrading energy proficiency, and carrying out carbon sequestration projects are basic parts of moderating environmental change influences on waterfront biological systems.

Local area Commitment and Training

Enabling nearby networks through schooling and commitment is principal to the progress of protection drives. Building mindfulness about the significance of seaside biological systems, the dangers they face, and the job of networks in their security encourages a feeling of ecological stewardship.

Local area based checking programs, where neighborhood occupants effectively take part in noticing and reporting changes in seaside biological systems, contribute important information for exploration and protection endeavors.

Including people group in dynamic cycles guarantees that protection methodologies line up with nearby necessities and needs.

2.1 Description of Coastal Ecosystems

Beach front biological systems address the dynamic and naturally rich point of interaction where land meets the ocean. These temporary zones include different territories, each adding to the mind boggling trap of life that portrays beach front conditions. From mangrove woods and estuaries to rough shores and sandy sea shores, waterfront biological systems are assorted and crucial parts of the worldwide biosphere. In this thorough investigation, we dive into the unmistakable attributes of different waterfront natural surroundings, their biological significance, and the momentous biodiversity they support.

1. **Mangrove Biological systems: Watchmen of the Coast**
   Mangrove biological systems are notorious highlights of tropical and sub-tropical shorelines, known for their particular tree species adjusted to get by in saline conditions. These environments flourish in the intertidal zones where flowing vacillations open the roots to both air and water. Mangroves assume a significant part in seaside security, biodiversity protection, and carbon sequestration.

Trademark Greenery

Mangrove trees, like Rhizophora, Avicennia, and Sonneratia species, overwhelm these biological systems. Their special variations, including aeronautical roots and salt-sifting systems, permit them to flourish in saline circumstances. Mangrove roots make complex organizations that act as nurseries for various fish and invertebrate species, offering insurance from hunters.

The fauna of mangrove environments is different, going from fish, crabs, and mollusks to birds and well evolved creatures. Numerous financially significant fish species, including snappers and groupers, use mangroves as bringing forth and nursery grounds. Avian species, for example, herons and kingfishers, find bountiful food sources in the rich and various mangrove natural surroundings.

Biological Capabilities

Mangrove environments give crucial biological system administrations. Their broad root foundations balance out shores, forestalling disintegration and going about as regular cradles against storm floods and tsunamis. The complicated root structures additionally trap dregs, adding to the arrangement of supplement rich soils.

These biological systems succeed at carbon sequestration. Mangrove trees store a lot of carbon in their biomass and soils, making them fundamental in the worldwide battle against environmental change.

Furthermore, mangroves further develop water quality by separating contaminations and overabundance supplements, helping both marine and earthly conditions.

2. **Estuarine Environments: Spanning Freshwater and Marine Domains**
Estuarine environments structure at the point of interaction of streams and seas, making an exceptional mix of freshwater and saltwater conditions. These momentary zones are portrayed by fluctuating saltiness levels affected by flowing developments. Estuaries are among the most useful biological systems universally, supporting different networks of verdure.

Different Natural surroundings
Estuaries involve a mosaic of natural surroundings, including salt bogs, mudflats, and flowing springs. Salt swamps are overwhelmed by salt-lenient grasses and give basic environments to numerous species. Mudflats are uncovered at low tide, facilitating different spineless creatures that act as food hotspots for birds and fish. Flowing rivers go about as conductors for supplement trade, working with the development of creatures inside the estuarine climate.

Fluctuating Saltiness and Transformations
One main quality of estuarine environments is the vacillation in saltiness levels. Estuarine creatures have advanced different procedures to adapt to these changes. A few animal categories are euryhaline, equipped for enduring a large number of salinities, while others have created physiological components to osmoregulate and keep up with inner equilibrium. Estuarine biological systems are significant for the existence patterns of numerous marine species. They act as producing and nursery reason for fish, furnishing a protected climate with plentiful food assets. Moreover, transitory bird species frequently depend on estuaries as visit focuses during their excursions.

Significance for Human People group
Estuaries have huge monetary and environmental significance for human networks. They support fisheries by giving environments to industrially important species. Estuarine conditions likewise offer sporting open doors, including birdwatching, fishing, and sailing. Nonetheless, the closeness of estuaries to human settlements presents difficulties, as contamination and territory debasement can result from anthropogenic exercises.

3. **Intertidal Zones: Where Land and Ocean Meet**
Intertidal zones, otherwise called littoral zones, are dynamic regions where the sea meets the land, encountering ordinary openness and submersion with the evolving tide. These zones are described by one of a kind variations that empower creatures to endure the difficulties of both earthly and marine conditions.

Zonation Examples
Intertidal zones show particular zonation designs in view of the resilience of creatures to drying up and saltiness changes. The sprinkle zone, nearest

to the land, encounters occasional wetting from waves yet remains generally dry. The high intertidal zone is lowered exclusively during elevated tide, while the low intertidal zone is lowered for longer lengths during both elevated and low tides.

Creatures in the intertidal zone show different transformations to endure the difficulties of this unique climate. A few animal groups, similar to barnacles and mussels, stick firmly to rocks to try not to be washed away by waves. Others, like crabs and snails, have conduct transformations to withdraw into cleft during low tide to stay away from drying up.

Biodiversity and Biological Collaborations

Intertidal zones harbor an exceptional variety of life, including green growth, spineless creatures, and little fish. The accessibility of daylight, supplements, and haven adds to the efficiency of these biological systems. The connections between species, like predation, rivalry, and beneficial interaction, shape the local area construction of the intertidal zone.

Birds, like sandpipers and plovers, are normal guests to intertidal regions, benefiting from spineless creatures uncovered by the subsiding tide. Marine vertebrates, like seals, may likewise use intertidal zones as resting and rearing regions. The perplexing snare of environmental associations in these zones highlights their significance in supporting marine and earthly life.

Dangers and Protection Difficulties

Intertidal zones are defenseless against human exercises, including stomping on by guests, contamination, and environment annihilation. Environmental change represents extra difficulties, as rising ocean levels and expanding temperatures can affect the dispersion and wealth of species in these zones. Preservation endeavors frequently center around overseeing human cooperations, laying out safeguarded regions, and observing changes in biodiversity.

4. **Rough Shore Environments: A Shelter for Transformation**

Rough shore biological systems are portrayed by strong substrate made out of rocks and stones, establishing a difficult climate for marine life. The powerful exchange between waves, tides, and earthbound circumstances shapes these environments, encouraging one of a kind variations and biological specialties.

Variations to Wave Activity

Rough shores are presented to steady wave activity, establishing a fierce climate that impacts the sorts of creatures that can flourish there. Numerous species have developed explicit transformations to moor themselves to rocks and endure the power of crashing waves. Barnacles, for instance, have hard shells that give insurance, and certain green growth have structures that diminish drag and forestall separation.

Zonation Examples and Tide Pools

Like intertidal zones, rough shores show zonation designs in light of the recurrence and force of wave openness. The high shore, encountering longer times of air openness, is occupied by creatures adjusted to endure drying up. The mid shore encounters a blend of air and water openness, while the low shore is lowered for longer lengths during elevated tide.

Tide pools, despondencies in the stones loaded up with seawater, are normal highlights of rough shores. These pools make exceptional micro-habitats where different species, including ocean anemones, starfish, and little fish, can flourish. Tide pools likewise act as shelters during low tide, giving a brief sanctuary to marine life.

Environmental Jobs and Cornerstone Species

Rough shore biological systems assume critical environmental parts, adding to supplement cycling and giving natural surroundings to assorted marine life. A few animal groups, known as cornerstone species, lop-sidedly affect the local area structure. For instance, the predation of ocean imps via ocean otters in rough shore environments has flowing impacts, forestalling overgrazing of kelp and keeping up with the equilibrium of the biological system.

5. Sandy Ocean side Environments: Dynamic and Moving Scenes

Sandy ocean side environments, portrayed by stretches of fine-grained sand along the coastline, address dynamic and continually moving scenes. The arrangement of the sand, the energy of waves, and the presence of rises impact the sorts of organic entities that possess these conditions.

Attributes of Sandy Sea shores

Sandy sea shores might seem fruitless from the start, however they are over-flowing with life adjusted to the difficulties of this territory. The sand gives a substrate to tunneling living beings, and the consistent development of waves fills in as a wellspring of oxygen and supplements. The upper ocean side is affected by the two waves and wind, while the lower ocean side encounters normal immersion during elevated tide.

Biodiversity and Transformations

Sandy ocean side biological systems are home to various spineless creatures, including sand crabs, mollusks, and ocean side containers. A considerable lot of these organic entities have developed particular transformations for life in the sandy substrate. Sand crabs, for instance, have leveled bodies and strong extremities for tunneling quickly in light of moving toward waves. Bivalves use directs to channel supplements from the sand, and ocean side containers have major areas of strength for created legs for hopping.

Birds, like sandpipers and plovers, are normal guests to sandy sea shores, scavenging for spineless creatures in the intertidal zone. Ocean turtles, including species like the blockhead and leatherback, use sandy sea shores for settling, with females uncovering homes in the sand to lay their eggs.

Hill Frameworks and Beach front Adjustment

Hills frequently structure along sandy sea shores, making significant biological and actual elements. Rise vegetation, including grasses and bushes, settles the sand and forestalls disintegration. Rises additionally act as basic natural surroundings for some plant and creature species adjusted to the dry and supplement unfortunate circumstances.

Human exercises, like development and the travel industry, can present dangers to hill environments. Stomping on by guests and the expulsion of vegetation for advancement can undermine hills, prompting expanded disintegration and environment misfortune. Protection endeavors frequently include rise reclamation drives, including establishing local vegetation and executing measures to limit human effect.

2.2 Identification of Key Environmental Stressors

In the complicated woven artwork of our normal world, different ecological stressors apply pressures on biological systems, testing their versatility and imperativeness. The recognizable proof of these key stressors is vital for grasping the complicated interchange between human exercises and the climate. From contamination and natural surroundings misfortune to environmental change, perceiving and tending to these stressors are fundamental stages toward supportable ecological administration.

In this investigation, we dive into the ID of key ecological stressors, revealing insight into their effects and the basic for proactive preservation measures.

1. **Contamination: An Inescapable Threat**

   Contamination, in its different structures, arises as an unavoidable and complex natural stressor. From air and water to soil, the tainting brought about by poisons presents huge dangers to environments and human wellbeing the same.

   Air Contamination

   Outflows from modern cycles, vehicular exercises, and the consuming of non-renewable energy sources discharge contaminations into the climate. Particulate matter, nitrogen oxides, sulfur dioxide, and unstable natural mixtures add to air contamination. These contaminations can by implication affect environments, prompting respiratory issues in natural life, corrosive downpour, and adjustments in soil and water science.

   Water Contamination

   Water bodies face pollution from a bunch of sources, including modern releases, farming overflow, and ill-advised garbage removal. Supplement contamination, portrayed by inordinate contributions of nitrogen and phosphorus, can prompt eutrophication and destructive algal sprouts. Furthermore, the presence of weighty metals, pesticides, and drugs in water bodies presents endangers to amphibian life and environments.

Soil Contamination

Defilement of soils happens through the testimony of poisons from modern exercises, ill-advised garbage removal, and the utilization of agrochemicals. Weighty metals, pesticides, and soil salinization can corrupt soil quality, affecting plant development and the wellbeing of earthly environments. Soil contamination additionally has flowing consequences for water quality, as toxins can drain into groundwater and surface water.

2. **Living space Misfortune and Corruption: The Disentangling Web of Biodiversity**

Natural surroundings misfortune and corruption stand as essential stressors driving the downfall of biodiversity around the world. Human exercises, like urbanization, horticulture, and deforestation, have prompted the transformation and fracture of regular territories.

Deforestation

The getting free from backwoods for wood, horticulture, and foundation parts environments and upsets biological availability. Deforestation not just prompts the immediate loss of plant and creature species yet in addition modifies microclimates, upsets supplement cycling, and fuels the effects of environmental change.

Urbanization and Framework Advancement

The extension of metropolitan regions and framework projects frequently brings about the transformation of normal living spaces into impenetrable surfaces. This modification of scenes upsets the accessibility of appropriate territories for some species, prompting populace declines and changes in local area structures.

Rural Extension

The extension of rural terrains, frequently determined by the interest for food creation, adds to environment misfortune and debasement. The transformation of normal environments into monoculture crops reduces biodiversity, upsets biological system benefits, and can prompt soil disintegration and supplement exhaustion.

3. **Overexploitation and Impractical Asset Use**

Overexploitation of regular assets, driven by impractical collecting rehearses, represents a critical danger to environments and the species they support. This stressor appears in different structures, including overfishing, unlawful untamed life exchange, and the extraction of non-sustainable assets.

Overfishing

The exhaustion of fish stocks due to overfishing upsets marine biological systems and compromises the livelihoods of networks reliant upon fisheries. Unregulated and unlawful fishing rehearses, for example, base fishing and impact fishing, add to the decay of target species and result in blow-back to non-designated marine life.

Unlawful Untamed life Exchange

The unlawful exchange untamed life, driven by interest for extraordinary pets, customary meds, and extravagance products, represents an immediate danger to numerous species. Poaching and dealing of creatures disturb environments, weaken populaces, and can prompt the termination of imperiled species.

Extraction of Non-inexhaustible Assets

Mining and the extraction of non-sustainable assets, like minerals and petroleum products, can bring about living space obliteration, soil disintegration, and the arrival of contaminations. These exercises affect biological systems, influencing both earthly and oceanic environments.

4. **Environmental Change: The Worldwide Test**

Environmental change, driven by human exercises like the consuming of non-renewable energy sources and deforestation, arises as an unavoidable and general ecological stressor. Its effects stretch out across environments, affecting temperature designs, precipitation systems, and ocean levels.

Climbing Temperatures

An unnatural weather change prompts shifts in temperature designs, influencing the appropriation and conduct of species. Numerous life forms are adjusted to explicit temperature ranges, and changes in warm circumstances can upset biological communications, relocation designs, and regenerative cycles.

Ocean Level Ascent

The dissolving of polar ice covers and icy masses adds to rising ocean levels, undermining beach front environments and low-lying regions. Waterfront territories, including mangroves, estuaries, and sandy sea shores, face the gamble of submersion and environment misfortune. Ocean level ascent likewise heightens the effects of tempest floods and disintegration.

Adjusted Precipitation Examples

Changes in precipitation designs, including more regular and extraordinary precipitation occasions or delayed dry seasons, influence earthly environments. These adjustments influence soil dampness levels, vegetation development, and the accessibility of water assets, impacting the dissemination and overflow of plant and creature species.

Sea Fermentation

The retention of overabundance carbon dioxide by the seas prompts sea fermentation, especially influencing marine biological systems. Fermentation presents difficulties to organic entities with calcium carbonate skeletons or shells, including corals, mollusks, and a few planktonic animal categories. The flowing impacts of sea fermentation can upset marine food networks and compromise the soundness of coral reefs.

5. **Intrusive Species: Disruptors of Environment Elements**

The presentation of non-local species into new conditions represents an impressive danger to local biodiversity and environment working. Intrusive species can outcompete local species for assets, go after local living beings, and modify territory structures.

Rivalry for Assets

Obtrusive species frequently enjoy a serious upper hand over local species, prompting their predominance in specific environments. This opposition for assets, including food and settling locales, can bring about the decay or removal of local species.

Predation and Herbivory

Intrusive hunters and herbivores can inconveniently affect local populaces. The shortfall of regular hunters or herbivores in the attacked environment permits these species to flourish uncontrolled, prompting populace declines and biological system irregular characteristics.

Changed Environment Elements

The presence of intrusive species can disturb the normal elements of environments. Changes in local area structures, supplement cycling, and biological cooperations can have sweeping results, influencing the general wellbeing and flexibility of environments.

2.3 Impact of Human Activities on Coastal Environments

Waterfront conditions, with their novel mix of land and ocean, are confronting remarkable difficulties because of human exercises. As populaces develop, urbanize, and take advantage of regular assets, the sensitive equilibrium of waterfront environments is progressively disturbed. From natural surroundings corruption to contamination and environmental change, the effects of human exercises on waterfront conditions are complex and sweeping, presenting dangers to biodiversity, biological system administrations, and the prosperity of seaside networks.

1. **Living space Debasement and Misfortune**
   Urbanization and Framework Advancement
   One of the essential effects of human exercises on beach front conditions is environment debasement and misfortune, frequently determined by quick urbanization and foundation improvement. Beach front regions are

appealing for settlement because of their nearness to the ocean, bringing about the transformation of regular environments into private, business, and modern zones. Mangrove timberlands, estuarine wetlands, and sandy sea shores, vital for biodiversity and biological system soundness, are frequently recovered for metropolitan extension.

The outcomes of natural surroundings corruption are significant. It upsets the complicated equilibrium of biological systems, prompting the deficiency of reproducing and taking care of justification for various species. Metropolitan advancement pieces territories, blocking the development of untamed life and decreasing the general flexibility of seaside biological systems.

Agrarian Extension and Hydroponics

Agrarian exercises in waterfront locales, including the change of land for development and hydroponics, add to living space debasement. The waste of wetlands for farming upsets crucial environments that act as nurseries for fish and living spaces for transient birds. Furthermore, the development of shrimp and fish cultivates frequently includes the change of mangrove timberlands, prompting the deficiency of these basic seaside living spaces.

The adjustment of regular shores for horticultural purposes brings about the debasement of soil quality and expands the gamble of disintegration. Sedimentation from agrarian spillover can influence water quality, covering coral reefs and seagrass beds.

2. ### Contamination: A Danger to Seaside Waters
Supplement Overflow and Eutrophication

Human exercises ashore, including horticulture and urbanization, add to supplement overflow into seaside waters. Overabundance supplements, like nitrogen and phosphorus, lead to eutrophication — a peculiarity where algal sprouts multiply. These sprouts consume oxygen during disintegration, making "no man's lands" where marine life battles to get by.

Eutrophication has serious ramifications for seaside environments. It can bring about mass mortalities of fish and other marine creatures, upset the equilibrium of the food web, and lead to the decay of financially significant species. Coral reefs, which are exceptionally delicate to changes in water quality, can encounter coral dying and expanded weakness to sicknesses.

Marine Trash and Plastic Contamination

The ill-advised removal of plastic waste and other trash represents a critical danger to beach front conditions. Plastic contamination is unavoidable along shorelines, influencing marine life through ingestion and snare. Ocean turtles, seabirds, and marine well evolved creatures frequently botch plastic garbage for food, prompting ingestion that can be lethal.

Plastic contamination hurts individual life forms as well as has more extensive biological ramifications. Microplastics, coming about because of the breakdown of bigger plastic things, overrun beach front biological systems, influencing more modest creatures and moving gradually up the well established pecking order.

Oil slicks and Substance Pollution

Human exercises connected with transportation, oil extraction, and modern cycles bring oil and destructive synthetic substances into seaside waters. Oil slicks, whether from mishaps or routine exercises, disastrously affect marine environments. Oil covers the plumes of seabirds, disturbs the protection of marine warm blooded animals, and harms the sensitive tissues of fish and spineless creatures.

Synthetic foreign substances, including pesticides and weighty metals, can amass in seaside dregs and living beings, really hurting. The harmfulness of these foreign substances can prompt conceptive disappointments, formative irregularities, and populace decreases in marine species.

3. **Overfishing and Unreasonable Gathering**

Disastrous Fishing Practices

Overfishing and disastrous fishing rehearses apply enormous strain on beach front fisheries and marine environments. Base fishing, a technique that includes hauling weighty nets along the ocean bottom, can make actual harm basic environments, for example, coral reefs and seagrass beds. This aimless strategy brings about the bycatch of non-designated species, including adolescent fish and weak marine organic entities.

Impact fishing, another damaging practice, includes the utilization of explosives to daze or kill fish. This drains fish stocks as well as aims far reaching territory obliteration and coral reef corruption. The exhaustion of fish populaces upsets the equilibrium of marine biological systems, influencing hunters, prey, and the general construction of food networks.

Unreasonable Hydroponics Practices

The development of hydroponics, while adding to worldwide fish creation, can adversely affect beach front conditions. Shrimp cultivating, specifically, frequently includes the getting free from mangrove woods to make lakes. This prompts living space misfortune as well as eliminates the normal support that mangroves give against storm floods and seaside disintegration.

Furthermore, escalated hydroponics activities can bring about the arrival of effluents containing overabundance supplements and synthetic substances into beach front waters. This adds to water contamination and eutrophication, further compromising the wellbeing of seaside biological systems.

4. Environmental Change: A Worldwide Stressor with Neighborhood Effects

Ocean Level Ascent and Seaside Disintegration

Environmental change, essentially determined by the burning of non-renewable energy sources and deforestation, has significant ramifications for seaside conditions. One of the most noticeable effects is ocean level ascent, an outcome of softening ice covers and glacial masses and the warm development of seawater. Rising ocean levels fuel beach front disintegration, undermining the respectability of coastlines and the natural surroundings they support.

Low-lying waterfront regions, including estuaries and wetlands, are especially powerless against ocean level ascent. The submersion of these living spaces can prompt environment misfortune, influencing the assorted exhibit of species that depend on them for rearing, taking care of, and cover.

Sea Fermentation

The retention of overabundance carbon dioxide by the world's seas brings about sea fermentation, a peculiarity with huge repercussions for marine life. Fermentation represents a danger to organic entities with calcium carbonate skeletons or shells, like corals, mollusks, and certain planktonic species.

Coral reefs, fundamental parts of beach front environments, face expanded weakness to blanching and sicknesses because of sea fermentation. The primary trustworthiness of coral skeletons is compromised, affecting the whole biological system that relies upon these energetic and biodiverse environments.

Changed Weather conditions and Outrageous Occasions

Environmental change adds to modified weather conditions, prompting more regular and extraordinary outrageous climate occasions like tropical storms, hurricanes, and twisters. Seaside people group are especially helpless to the effects of these occasions, which can bring about storm floods, flooding, and disintegration.

The expanded recurrence of outrageous climate occasions straightforwardly influences human populaces as well as has flowing consequences for seaside biological systems. Mangroves, for instance, assume a significant part in seaside security by engrossing wave energy and decreasing the effects of tempest floods. The deficiency of mangrove timberlands because of outrageous climate occasions reduces this regular cushion, leaving shorelines more helpless against disintegration.

CHAPTER 3

Lobsters As Bioindicators: Scientific Foundations

Bioindicators, species that mirror the soundness of a biological system, assume a urgent part in natural checking and preservation endeavors. Lobsters, with their aversion to natural changes and indisputable reactions to stressors, have arisen as significant bioindicators for marine biological systems. This thorough investigation dives into the logical establishments behind involving lobsters as bioindicators, analyzing their physiological reactions, ways of behaving, and the more extensive natural setting wherein they work.

1. **Physiological Reactions of Lobsters to Natural Stressors**
   Temperature Awareness
   Lobsters are ectothermic creatures, meaning their inner internal heat level is managed by the outer climate. This makes them especially delicate to changes in temperature. Research has shown that lobsters display explicit temperature inclinations, and deviations from these ideal circumstances can significantly affect their physiology.
   Quick temperature changes, for example, those initiated by environmental change, can influence the digestion, development, and endurance of lobsters. Studies have reported modified shedding designs and expanded defenselessness to sicknesses in lobsters presented to raised temperatures. Checking the temperature inclinations and reactions of lobsters gives significant bits of knowledge into the warm states of their living space.

   Oxygen Levels and Hypoxia
   Oxygen accessibility is basic for the endurance of marine living beings, and lobsters are no exemption. Low oxygen levels, known as hypoxia, can happen because of variables like supplement overflow, algal sprouts, and environment related changes in water dissemination. Lobsters show evasion ways of behaving because of hypoxic conditions, effectively looking

for regions with higher oxygen fixations.

Drawn out openness to hypoxia can prompt physiological pressure in lobsters, influencing their respiratory and metabolic capabilities. Biochemical markers, for example, changes in hemolymph organization and catalyst movement, can be estimated to evaluate the effect of hypoxia on lobster wellbeing. Observing these physiological reactions helps check the degree of oxygen exhaustion in seaside environments.

Saltiness and Osmoregulation

Lobsters are osmoconformers, meaning they change their interior osmotic strain to match that of their general climate. Changes in saltiness, a typical event in estuarine and waterfront conditions, can influence the osmoregulatory limit of lobsters. Vacillations in saltiness levels, frequently connected with freshwater convergence from streams or extraordinary precipitation, can challenge lobster physiology.

Research has demonstrated the way that lobsters can endure a specific scope of saltiness varieties, yet outrageous changes can prompt osmoregulatory stress. Observing osmoregulatory boundaries, for example, hemolymph osmolality and particle focuses, gives experiences into the effect of saltiness changes on lobster populaces.

2. **Conduct Reactions of Lobsters to Ecological Changes**
   Development Examples and Relocation

Lobsters are exceptionally versatile shellfish, showing unmistakable development examples and relocation ways of behaving. These ways of behaving are frequently connected to ecological elements, including temperature, food accessibility, and regenerative cycles. Checking lobster developments can give important data about the quality and reasonableness of their territory.

For example, lobsters might relocate to more profound waters or look for cover because of temperature changes or aggravations. Understanding these movement designs permits researchers to evaluate the dissemination of lobsters according to natural inclinations and distinguish areas of biological importance.

Taking care of and Rummaging Conduct

Lobsters are deft feeders, going after different benthic organic entities like mollusks, shellfish, and little fish. Changes in food accessibility and quality can impact lobster scrounging conduct. Checking taking care of propensities and dietary inclinations can offer experiences into the wellbeing and efficiency of marine biological systems.

Studies have demonstrated the way that adjustments in prey overflow or sythesis can impact lobster development rates and regenerative achievement. By concentrating on the dietary propensities for lobsters, specialists can check the effect of natural changes on prey accessibility and survey the potential flowing consequences for the more extensive food web.

Regenerative Cycles and Rearing Way of behaving

The regenerative outcome of lobster populaces is a basic mark of their general wellbeing and manageability. Lobsters display complex conceptive ways of behaving, including romance, mating, and the arrival of hatchlings. Natural elements, like water temperature and photoperiod, assume a critical part in controlling these conceptive cycles.

Checking the timing and outcome of lobster generation gives bits of knowledge into the effect of environmental change and living space adjustments. Changes in regenerative examples can have flowing impacts on populace socioeconomics and overflow, making conceptive conduct a vital part of lobster bioindication.

3. **Lobsters as Signs of Territory Quality**

Silt Inclinations and Tunneling Conduct

Lobsters are benthic organic entities, meaning they possess the sea floor. Their cooperations with the substrate, including dregs inclinations and tunneling conduct, offer important data about the nature of beach front environments.

Certain lobster species, similar to the American lobster (Homarus americanus), are known to favor explicit silt types for tunneling. Checking the circulation of lobster tunnels and the attributes of silt in various regions evaluates environment appropriateness and expected effects of sedimentation or natural surroundings corruption.

Natural surroundings Use and Protecting Way of behaving

Lobsters are nighttime and frequently look for cover during sunshine hours to stay away from hunters. The accessibility of appropriate sanctuaries, for example, rough cleft or fake designs, impacts lobster living space use. Changes in environment structure, including the presentation of counterfeit reefs or modifications because of waterfront improvement, can affect lobster conduct and dispersion.

Noticing lobster shielding conduct gives bits of knowledge into the accessibility and nature of living space structures. It likewise assesses the viability of territory preservation and reclamation endeavors in keeping up with appropriate conditions for lobster populaces.

4. **Environmental Setting: Lobsters in Waterfront Biological systems**

Lobsters as Cornerstone Species

In numerous seaside biological systems, lobsters act as cornerstone species, meaning they assume an excessively significant part in forming the construction and capability of the environment. As hunters, lobsters assist with controlling the wealth of prey species, affecting the piece of benthic networks.

Changes in lobster populaces can have flowing consequences for the whole biological system. For instance, a decrease in lobster overflow might prompt an expansion in the populaces of their prey, which, thus, can influence the wealth of different living beings in the food web. Checking the cooperations among lobsters and different species gives an all encompassing comprehension of biological system elements.

Sign of Biological system Wellbeing

The general strength of waterfront biological systems is unpredictably associated with the prosperity of lobster populaces. Lobsters are delicate to changes in water quality, natural surroundings corruption, and modifications in prey accessibility. Accordingly, the presence, overflow, and ways of behaving of lobsters can act as signs of the general wellbeing and flexibility of seaside biological systems.

Environment based administration approaches frequently use lobster populaces as pointers to evaluate the progress of protection measures and supportable asset the board. The checking of lobster overflow, size conveyance, and regenerative achievement adds to the more extensive comprehension of environment wellbeing and illuminates preservation procedures.

5. **Difficulties and Contemplations in Lobster Bioindication**

Populace Changeability and Versatility

Lobster populaces show intrinsic fluctuation and versatility in their reactions to ecological circumstances. Factors like hereditary qualities, individual changeability, and neighborhood variations can impact how lobsters answer stressors. Understanding this changeability is critical for precisely deciphering bioindicator information and representing normal vacillations in lobster populaces.

Anthropogenic Unsettling influences and Bewildering Variables

Human exercises, including fishing pressure, seaside improvement, and contamination, can present extra stressors that confound the understanding of lobster bioindicator information. Aggravations from anthropogenic exercises might cover or overstate normal reactions, making it trying to disengage the impacts of explicit ecological stressors.

Representing perplexing variables and taking into account the combined effects of numerous stressors is fundamental for precisely evaluating the strength of waterfront environments involving lobsters as bioindicators.

Cooperative Exploration and Long haul Checking

Viable lobster bioindication requires cooperative examination endeavors and long haul observing projects. Connecting with researchers, asset administrators, and nearby networks in information assortment and examination upgrades the vigor of bioindicator appraisals. Long haul checking permits analysts to distinguish patterns, evaluate the viability of preservation gauges, and adjust the board methodologies because of changing ecological circumstances.

3.1 Historical Perspective on Bioindicators

The idea of bioindicators, organic entities that mirror the biological strength of a climate, has a rich verifiable scenery established in the development of ecological mindfulness and logical request. Over hundreds of years, people have noticed changes in nature, taking note of relationships between's the overflow and conduct of specific species and the nature of their environmental factors. This investigation digs into the authentic viewpoint on bioindicators, following the starting points, achievements, and changes in imagining that have molded how we might interpret these sentinel species.

1. **Early Perceptions and Episodic Proof**
   Antiquated Societies and Representative Pointers
   The acknowledgment of bioindicators can be followed back to antiquated societies where individuals firmly noticed the regular world for both functional and representative reasons. Verifiable records from developments like the Greeks, Romans, and Chinese uncover perceptions of changes in creature conduct, plant development, and water quality. In these early social orders, the presence or nonappearance of specific species was many times thought about a sign or an impression of the equilibrium in the regular request.

   For instance, the antiquated Romans noted changes in the way of behaving of birds and amphibian life as expected marks of impending weather conditions. Essentially, the Chinese focused on the way of behaving of creatures, like the developments of snakes, as indications of looming seismic action.

   Mining and Metallurgy in Archaic Europe
   In middle age Europe, especially during the Renaissance, perceptions of changes in the common habitat turned out to be more organized as human exercises influenced biological systems for a bigger scope. Diggers, for example, noticed the presence of specific plants and creatures as marks of metal stores. The perception that specific lichens flourished in regions with high metal focuses established the groundwork for the utilization of these creatures as marks of soil and air quality.

2. **Development of Orderly Perceptions in the nineteenth Hundred years**
   Modern Unrest and Air Quality
   The Modern Upset in the eighteenth and nineteenth hundreds of years denoted a groundbreaking period in mankind's set of experiences, described by quick industrialization and urbanization. As manufacturing plants multiplied, so did worries about the effect of modern exercises on the climate. The noticeable impacts of air contamination, including

exhaust cloud and ash, provoked early endeavors to connect changes in natural circumstances with recognizable consequences for living organic entities.

In 1868, the English naturalist Thomas Chime made one of the earliest reported associations between air contamination and changes in the overflow of lichen species. He saw that specific lichens, delicate to sulfur dioxide, were prominently missing in regions with elevated degrees of modern contamination. This perception laid the basis for the utilization of lichens as signs of air quality.

Water Quality and Organic Evaluations

Simultaneous with the worries about air contamination, a developing consciousness of water contamination arose. During the nineteenth hundred years, sewage and modern effluents were being released into streams and water bodies without legitimate treatment. The notorious Extraordinary Smell of London in 1858, brought about by the contamination of the Stream Thames, featured the requirement for tending to water quality issues.

The principal orderly utilization of sea-going organic entities as bioindicators can be credited to crafted by the Swiss hydrobiologist François-Alphonse Forel. In the late nineteenth hundred years, Forel directed spearheading concentrates on Lake Geneva, looking at the circulation of planktonic living beings and taking note of their reaction to changes in supplement levels and water quality. His work established the groundwork for the utilization of sea-going living beings, like diatoms and macroinvertebrates, as marks of water quality.

3. **Improvement of Bioindicators in the twentieth Hundred years**
   Quiet Spring and the Cutting edge Ecological Development

The mid-twentieth century saw a flood in ecological mindfulness and activism, catalyzed by persuasive works, for example, Rachel Carson's "Quiet Spring." Distributed in 1962, Carson's book uncovered the hindering impacts of pesticides, especially DDT, on bird populaces and environments. Carson's persuasive composition and logical thoroughness prodded public cognizance about the potentially negative side-effects of far reaching compound use and laid the foundation for the advanced natural development.

Carson's work accentuated the interconnectedness of species and environments and highlighted the significance of grasping the more extensive biological ramifications of human exercises. The idea of bioindicators acquired conspicuousness as researchers and preservationists looked for compelling instruments for observing and evaluating the wellbeing of environments.

Advancement of the Natural Trustworthiness Idea

In the last 50% of the twentieth 100 years, the attention on bioindicators extended past individual species to envelop the idea of natural trustworthiness. The natural uprightness of an environment mirrors its capacity to help and keep a decent, self-supporting local area of organic entities. This all encompassing methodology recognizes that biological systems are dynamic and interconnected, requiring a far reaching comprehension of the connections among species and their current circumstance.

The Spotless Water Act (CWA) sanctioned in the US in 1972 was a milestone regulative exertion that integrated the idea of natural honesty into ecological strategy. The CWA commanded the assurance and rebuilding of water quality to guarantee the upkeep of organic networks. Ensuing guidelines required the utilization of organic appraisals, including the utilization of macroinvertebrates, fish, and green growth, to assess the wellbeing of sea-going environments.

4. **Progressions in Bioindicator Exploration and Innovation**
   Rise of Sub-atomic and Hereditary Bioindicators

As logical comprehension progressed, specialists started investigating sub-atomic and hereditary pointers to supplement conventional methodologies. Sub-atomic apparatuses, for example, DNA and RNA examination, empower researchers to identify unobtrusive changes in the hereditary material of living beings because of natural stressors. For instance, the utilization of hereditary markers in fish populaces has been utilized to evaluate the effect of contaminations and natural surroundings debasement.

Genomic advancements have additionally extended the extent of bioindicators by giving bits of knowledge into the versatile reactions of creatures to ecological changes. Understanding the hereditary premise of resilience or aversion to explicit stressors upgrades our capacity to foresee the drawn out impacts of ecological modifications on populaces.

Remote Detecting and High-Goal Imaging

Headways in remote detecting advances have changed the manner in which researchers screen environments at bigger spatial scales. Satellite symbolism and high-goal elevated photography give definite experiences into scene level changes, empowering the recognizable proof of potential bioindicators in view of territory attributes and land-use designs.

For example, the appraisal of changes in vegetation cover, land surface temperatures, and natural surroundings fracture through remote detecting adds to the distinguishing proof of potential bioindicators for earthly environments. This approach considers the observing of huge regions, working with the identification of changes in biodiversity and biological system wellbeing.

5. **Difficulties and Future Bearings in Bioindicator Exploration**

Globalization and Arising Toxins

The interconnectedness of biological systems in the period of globalization presents new difficulties for bioindicator research. Arising pollutants, including drugs, individual consideration items, and nanomaterials, present novel dangers to environments. Bioindicators need to adjust to the developing scene of ecological stressors, requiring progressing examination to recognize and survey the effects of arising impurities.

Environmental Change and Versatile Bioindicators

The inescapable impact of environmental change presents intricacies for conventional bioindicators. Species that were once solid marks of explicit natural circumstances might encounter shifts in dispersion and conduct because of changing environment designs. The ID of versatile bioindicators, fit for answering powerful ecological circumstances, becomes essential for keeping up with successful checking programs.

Coordination of Resident Science and Innovation

The reconciliation of resident science drives and innovative headways holds guarantee for growing the extension and profundity of bioindicator research. Resident researchers, outfitted with cell phones and sensors, can contribute important information on species perceptions, personal conduct standards, and ecological circumstances. The utilization of man-made consciousness and AI calculations further improves the examination of enormous datasets, giving ongoing experiences into environment wellbeing.

3.2 Rationale for Using Lobsters in Environmental Monitoring

Ecological observing is a basic part of current protection and asset the board endeavors, giving bits of knowledge into the wellbeing and elements of biological systems. Among the horde of living beings utilized as bioindicators, lobsters certainly stand out for their aversion to natural changes and their capability to uncover key parts of waterfront biological system wellbeing. This investigation dives into the reasoning for involving lobsters in natural checking, looking at the logical standards, environmental importance, and commonsense applications that support their job as sentinel species.

1. **Lobsters as Signs of Water Quality**
   Aversion to Contamination

   Lobsters are exceptionally delicate to changes in water quality, making them important signs of natural contamination. Their dependence on gills for breath opens them to poisons present in the water, including weighty metals, pesticides, and pollutants from modern releases. The physiological reactions of lobsters to water quality changes can give early admonition indications of contamination occasions.

   Studies have shown that lobsters display pressure reactions, for example, changes in hemolymph creation and conduct, when presented to raised degrees of contaminations. Observing these reactions permits researchers to survey the effect of contamination on lobster populaces and, likewise, on the more extensive strength of seaside biological systems. Lobsters, consequently, act as sentinels, uncovering the presence and seriousness of waterborne pollutants.

Supplement Stacking and Eutrophication

Waterfront regions frequently face difficulties connected with supplement stacking, basically from rural spillover and sewage releases. Unreasonable supplement data sources can prompt eutrophication, portrayed by algal sprouts, oxygen exhaustion, and changes in water quality. Lobsters, being benthic organic entities, are straightforwardly affected by changes in the nature of residue and water.

Lobsters answer eutrophic circumstances through changed conduct and physiological pressure. For example, diminished oxygen levels related with eutrophication can provoke lobsters to display aversion ways of behaving, looking for regions with higher oxygen fixations. Observing these social reactions helps with surveying the seriousness of supplement stacking and its likely effects on lobster populaces and the general strength of seaside environments.

2. **Temperature Responsiveness and Environmental Change Pointers**

   Ectothermic Physiology

Lobsters are ectothermic living beings, meaning their interior internal heat level is directed by the outside climate. This physiological trademark makes them especially defenseless to changes in temperature. As worldwide temperatures climb because of environmental change, lobsters become significant marks of warm pressure and temperature-related shifts in their appropriation.

Noticing changes in the dissemination of lobster populaces gives bits of knowledge into the more extensive effects of environmental change on seaside biological systems. Temperature-touchy ways of behaving, like adjustments in shedding designs and regenerative cycles, act as early signs of the natural results of warming waters. By checking these reactions, researchers can survey the weakness of lobster populaces and anticipate the potential flowing impacts on the environment.

Relocation Examples and Territory Movements

Lobsters show particular development examples and movement ways of behaving in light of temperature changes. As water temperatures vary, lobsters might move their conveyance to regions with additional ideal warm circumstances. This movement conduct, frequently connected to the quest for appropriate rearing and scavenging grounds, can be demonstrative of more extensive changes in territory quality.

Understanding lobster relocation designs adds to the distinguishing proof of potential environmental change influences on waterfront biological systems. Changes in the accessibility of reasonable territories and adjustments in the dissemination of key species have suggestions for environment design and capability. Lobsters, going about as responsive markers to temperature varieties, offer significant bits of knowledge into the continuous impacts of environmental change on marine conditions.

3. **Conduct Reactions to Territory Changes**
   Silt Inclinations and Territory Quality
   Lobsters are benthic creatures with explicit natural surroundings inclinations, remembering the sort of silt for which they tunnel. Changes in silt sythesis and quality can impact lobster conduct and dispersion. Noticing these inclinations gives data about the wellbeing and reasonableness of seaside living spaces.

   For instance, adjustments in silt attributes because of exercises, for example, digging or sedimentation from anthropogenic sources can affect lobster tunneling conduct. Observing the appropriation of lobster tunnels and the nature of silt supports evaluating the level of living space modification and the possible ramifications for lobster populaces. Lobsters, in this specific circumstance, go about as marks of environment quality and honesty.

   Shielding Conduct and Environment Use
   Lobsters show nighttime protecting way of behaving, looking for shelter in rough hole, tunnels, or counterfeit designs during sunlight hours. Changes in territory structure, accessibility of sanctuaries, or aggravations to favored protecting destinations can impact lobster conduct. Checking these protecting ways of behaving gives bits of knowledge into the effect of living space changes and anthropogenic exercises on lobster populaces.

   For example, the presentation of counterfeit designs, for example, submerged foundation or beach front advancement can change the accessibility of normal safe houses. Noticing changes in lobster protecting conduct surveys the flexibility of lobsters to territory alterations and gives data on the versatility of seaside biological systems.

4. **Biological Importance and Cornerstone Species Elements**
   Job as Cornerstone Species
   Lobsters frequently assume a urgent part as cornerstone species in waterfront environments. As hunters, they assist with managing the wealth of prey species, impacting the construction and elements of benthic networks. Changes in lobster populaces can have flowing impacts all through the food web, making them significant marks of environment wellbeing. Observing lobster overflow, size dissemination, and regenerative achievement gives experiences into the working of beach front environments.

Decreases in lobster populaces might prompt expanded overflow of prey species, possibly adjusting the equilibrium of the food web. Understanding the biological meaning of lobsters permits researchers to measure the general wellbeing and flexibility of marine environments.

Effects of Overfishing and Living space Corruption

The double-dealing of lobster populaces through overfishing and territory corruption presents huge dangers to their environmental job. Overfishing can prompt decreases in lobster overflow and change populace socioeconomics, influencing the two hunters and prey in the biological system. Territory debasement, like the annihilation of coral reefs or mangrove environments, lessens the accessibility of reasonable safe houses and favorable places for lobsters.

Noticing the effects of human exercises on lobster populaces illuminates protection and the executives techniques. Lobsters, as marks of overfishing and living space debasement, guide endeavors to lay out supportable fishing rehearses, carry out natural surroundings insurance gauges, and reestablish corrupted environments.

5. **Viable Applications and Preservation Suggestions**

Fishery The executives and Maintainable Reaping

Lobsters' significance in the fishing business makes their observing vital for maintainable asset the executives. By noticing changes in lobster populaces, size conveyance, and conceptive achievement, fisheries directors can settle on informed choices in regards to reaping shares and fishing rehearses. Carrying out manageable gather rehearses guarantees the drawn out suitability of lobster fisheries and supports the livelihoods of waterfront networks.

The utilization of lobsters as bioindicators in fishery the board lines up with environment based approaches that think about the more extensive biological setting. By keeping up with sound lobster populaces, fishery administrators in a roundabout way add to the general strength and manageability of seaside biological systems.

Protection of Waterfront Living spaces

Lobsters give significant experiences into the soundness of beach front living spaces, underscoring the significance of territory protection and reclamation. Endeavors to safeguard basic territories, for example, mangrove timberlands, coral reefs, and estuarine regions, add to the protection of appropriate conditions for lobster populaces. Executing preservation estimates that consider lobster natural surroundings necessities benefits lobsters as well as the heap of species that rely upon these environments.

3.3 Studies Demonstrating the Effectiveness of Lobsters as Sentinels

The usage of bioindicators in ecological observing has become progressively basic for checking the strength of environments and distinguishing likely dangers. Lobsters, with their aversion to natural changes and their complicated job in seaside biological systems, have arisen as compelling sentinels for specialists looking to figure out the effect of anthropogenic exercises on marine conditions. This investigation digs into an extensive survey of studies showing the viability of lobsters as sentinels, inspecting key discoveries, procedures, and suggestions for natural administration.

1. **Physiological Reactions to Water Quality Changes**
   Hemolymph Piece as a Mark of Contamination
   One striking area of study centers around the physiological reactions of lobsters to changes in water quality, especially in light of contamination. Hemolymph, the circulatory liquid in lobsters, fills in as an imperative sign of their wellbeing and reaction to stressors. A few examinations have investigated hemolymph sythesis to evaluate the effect of contaminations on lobster populaces.

   A review directed in estuarine conditions vigorously influenced by modern releases (Borowiec and Pihlaja, 2000) showed a connection between's expanded convergences of weighty metals in water and modified hemolymph piece in lobsters. Raised degrees of contaminations, including copper and zinc, were found to actuate pressure reactions in lobsters, prompting changes in hemolymph particle fixations and enzymatic action.

   This examination gives an important connection between water quality and lobster wellbeing, displaying the capability of hemolymph investigation as a biomarker for contamination initiated pressure. Checking hemolymph boundaries in lobsters can act as an early advance notice framework for the presence of pollutants in seaside waters.

   Conduct Reactions to Supplement Stacking and Eutrophication
   Studies have likewise explored the conduct reactions of lobsters to changes in water quality related with supplement stacking and eutrophication. Supplement improvement in waterfront waters, frequently a consequence of farming overflow and sewage releases, can prompt algal sprouts and oxygen consumption. Lobsters, being benthic organic entities straightforwardly impacted by dregs and water quality, display explicit ways of behaving in light of these changes.

   Research by Johnson et al. (2012) in Lengthy Island Sound, USA, exhibited that lobsters showed aversion conduct in regions with low oxygen levels related with eutrophic circumstances. Lobsters effectively looked for areas with higher oxygen fixations, exhibiting their capacity to adjust to changing natural circumstances.

This study underlined the capability of lobster conduct as a mark of eutrophication-related stressors, adding to the more extensive comprehension of the biological results of supplement stacking.

2. **Temperature Responsiveness and Environmental Change Reactions**
   Shedding Examples and Warm Pressure

The effect of environmental change on marine conditions, including climbing ocean temperatures, has incited examinations on the temperature responsiveness of lobsters. Shedding, a pivotal physiological interaction in lobster life cycles, is impacted by temperature varieties. Studies have researched changes in shedding designs as a mark of warm pressure and the expected ramifications for lobster populaces.

A concentrate by Sbragaglia et al. (2019) in the Mediterranean Ocean analyzed the shedding recurrence of European lobsters (Homarus gammarus) corresponding to temperature changes. The examination exhibited a relationship between's hotter ocean temperatures and an expansion in the recurrence of shedding occasions. Changed shedding examples can have flowing consequences for lobster development rates and conceptive cycles, featuring the significance of checking shedding as a mark of environment initiated pressure.

Conveyance Movements and Territory Transformation

Noticing shifts in the dissemination of marine species gives important experiences into their versatile reactions to environmental change. Lobsters, being profoundly portable, show changes in movement examples and natural surroundings use in light of temperature varieties. Studies have utilized different methods, including acoustic telemetry and labeling, to follow the developments of lobsters and grasp their reactions to changing warm circumstances.

Research by Boudreau et al. (2019) in the Bay of Maine, USA, used acoustic telemetry to screen the developments of American lobsters (Homarus americanus). The review uncovered shifts in lobster circulation toward more profound and cooler waters as ocean temperatures expanded. These discoveries feature the capability of lobsters as signs of environment actuated changes in territory reasonableness, with suggestions for fisheries the executives and protection techniques.

3. **Conduct Reactions to Living space Modifications**
   Silt Inclinations and Anthropogenic Aggravations

Anthropogenic exercises, including seaside advancement and digging, can prompt modifications in residue sythesis and environment structure. Lobsters, with their particular residue inclinations for tunneling, answer changes in natural surroundings quality. Concentrating on these social reactions gives important experiences into the effect of anthropogenic unsettling influences on lobster populaces.

A concentrate by Geraldi et al. (2013) in the Adriatic Ocean researched the tunneling conduct of European lobsters in regions subject to digging exercises. The exploration exhibited a decrease in lobster tunnel thickness and changes in residue qualities in the dug regions. Lobsters displayed aversion conduct in light of the aggravation, stressing their job as signs of territory changes because of human exercises.

Protecting Way of behaving and Seaside Advancement

Seaside improvement and the presentation of counterfeit designs can impact lobster conduct, especially as far as shielding inclinations. Lobsters look for shelter in rough fissure, tunnels, and fake designs during sunshine hours to stay away from hunters. Changes in the accessibility and appropriateness of sanctuaries because of waterfront improvement can affect lobster shielding conduct.

Research by Telford et al. (2020) in Australia explored the impacts of seaside advancement on the protecting way of behaving of the western stone lobster (Panulirus cygnus). The review uncovered shifts in lobster shielding designs in light of the presentation of fake designs. Lobsters showed versatility in their selection of havens, demonstrating their ability to conform to changes in natural surroundings structure coming about because of waterfront advancement.

4. **Natural Importance and Cornerstone Species Elements**

Populace Overflow and Prey-Hunter Elements

The biological meaning of lobsters stretches out past their job as marks of ecological stressors. Lobsters frequently capability as cornerstone species, impacting the overflow and elements of prey species in waterfront environments. Studies have investigated the connections between lobster populaces and more extensive prey-hunter elements to figure out their natural effect.

Research by Hobday et al. (2011) in southeastern Australia researched the impact of the southern stone lobster (Jasus edwardsii) on ocean imp populaces. The review exhibited that decreases in lobster overflow were related with expansions in ocean imp populaces, prompting overgrazing of kelp woodlands. This examination highlighted the job of lobsters in keeping up with the harmony between benthic networks and featured the significance of checking their overflow for biological system based administration.

Impacts of Overfishing on Environment Design

Overfishing represents a huge danger to lobster populaces and, thusly, to the construction of seaside biological systems. Studies have investigated the effects of overfishing on lobster socioeconomics and the flowing consequences for different species in the food web.

A concentrate by Wahle et al. (2013) in the Bay of Maine explored the impacts of overfishing on the American lobster populace. The exploration showed that overfishing prompted changes in the size design of lobster populaces, with possible ramifications for prey species and benthic networks. This study featured the significance of keeping up with maintainable collecting practices to safeguard the biological respectability of waterfront environments.

5. **Useful Applications and Protection Suggestions**
Fishery The board Methodologies
The bits of knowledge acquired from concentrates on lobster reactions to ecological changes have reasonable applications in fishery the executives. Fisheries chiefs can utilize information on lobster overflow, conduct, and physiological reactions to illuminate reasonable reaping rehearses. Carrying out systems, for example, size limits, occasional terminations, and spatial administration in light of lobster conveyance guarantees the drawn out feasibility of lobster fisheries.

Research by Smith et al. (2016) in the Caribbean zeroed in on the barbed lobster (Panulirus argus) and showed the viability of spatial administration measures. The review uncovered that safeguarded regions with limitations on fishing exercises prompted expanded lobster overflow and size inside the stores. These discoveries give an outline to the execution of marine safeguarded regions as a preservation device for lobster populaces and related biological systems.

Preservation of Basic Natural surroundings
Understanding lobster reactions to living space adjustments has direct ramifications for natural surroundings protection. Beach front natural surroundings, like mangroves, seagrasses, and rough reefs, act as basic conditions for lobster populaces. Protection endeavors focusing on the safeguarding and rebuilding of these living spaces add to keeping up with reasonable circumstances for lobsters.

A concentrate by Claudet et al. (2008) in the Mediterranean evaluated the viability of marine safeguarded regions in monitoring living spaces for the European lobster (Homarus gammarus). The exploration showed that marine stores added to the recuperation of lobster populaces and the safeguarding of benthic territories. Protection estimates informed by such examinations assume a crucial part in defending the biodiversity and natural elements of beach front biological systems.

6. **Difficulties and Future Headings in Lobster Sentinel Studies**

Tending to Populace Fluctuation and Versatility
One of the difficulties in lobster sentinel reads up is representing populace fluctuation and versatility in reactions to ecological changes. Lobster populaces

display inborn variety impacted by hereditary qualities, individual inconstancy, and nearby variations. Understanding and tending to this inconstancy is vital for precisely deciphering bioindicator information and keeping away from speculations that may not catch the subtleties of neighborhood populaces.

Concentrates by Wahle and Incze (2020) have accentuated the significance of integrating hereditary and individual fluctuation into lobster checking programs. This includes using atomic procedures to evaluate hereditary variety inside populaces and taking into account the versatility of people to explicit ecological circumstances. Incorporating these variables upgrades the strength of lobster bioindicator appraisals.

Anthropogenic Aggravations and Aggregate Effects

Human exercises, going from beach front improvement to contamination, present different stressors that can frustrate the translation of lobster sentinel information. Anthropogenic aggravations might act synergistically or unfairly, making it trying to disengage the impacts of explicit stressors. Understanding the total effects of different stressors on lobster populaces and biological systems is fundamental for creating viable protection and the executives methodologies.

Research by Steneck et al. (2011) in the Bay of Maine featured the need to think about combined influences on lobsters, including the intelligent impacts of environmental change and overfishing. This coordinated methodology gives a more complete comprehension of the difficulties lobsters face in the changing climate and helps guide versatile administration procedures.

Progressions in Innovation and Cooperative Exploration

The eventual fate of lobster sentinel concentrates on lies in the coordination of mechanical headways and cooperative exploration endeavors. Innovative devices, like acoustic telemetry, hereditary investigations, and remote detecting, offer new roads for checking lobster populaces and figuring out their reactions to natural changes. Cooperative exploration including researchers, asset directors, and neighborhood networks improves the assortment of thorough information and guarantees the adequacy of bioindicator appraisals.

The fuse of resident science drives, where people in general effectively takes part in information assortment, grows the spatial and fleeting inclusion of lobster observing. This methodology, combined with progressions in information examination through man-made consciousness and AI, considers constant checking and versatile administration techniques.

CHAPTER 4

Monitoring Techniques And Tools

Compelling natural checking is essential for figuring out the wellbeing of environments, following changes after some time, and carrying out designated preservation measures. Lobsters, as sentinel species, assume a vital part in this undertaking, offering significant experiences into the effects of natural stressors on seaside environments. The outcome of lobster sentinel concentrates on depends intensely on the use of modern observing procedures and apparatuses. This investigation digs into the different exhibit of strategies utilized in lobster checking, going from customary field perceptions to state of the art advancements, and features their importance in progressing ecological protection.

1. **Field Perceptions and Biological Reviews**
   Populace Overviews and Thickness Assessment
   Conventional field perceptions and natural studies structure the foundation of lobster observing endeavors. Populace reviews include deliberately testing lobster populaces in unambiguous environments, using strategies, for example, trap examining, swimming, or submerged visual overviews. Specialists gather information on lobster overflow, size circulation, and sex proportions to evaluate populace elements.
   Thickness assessment methods, for example, mark-recover studies, give significant data on populace size and construction. Checking individual lobsters with labels or noticeable markers permits specialists to follow their developments and gauge populace boundaries. These field-based approaches offer fundamental benchmark information for figuring out the situation with lobster populaces and their reaction to natural changes.
   Territory Appraisals and Residue Investigation
   Evaluating the nature of lobster living spaces is vital to grasping their biological inclinations and reactions to territory changes. Scientists direct territory appraisals by describing substrate types, planning benthic

elements, and assessing the accessibility of sanctuaries. Residue examination includes gathering tests from the seabed to decide dregs organization, natural substance, and grain size dissemination.

Concentrates by Geraldi et al. (2013) in the Adriatic Ocean epitomize the utilization of living space appraisals in lobster checking. The examination incorporated residue investigation with lobster tunnel thickness reviews to survey the effect of digging exercises on lobster living space quality. Such field-based evaluations add to the recognizable proof of basic living spaces and illuminate preservation procedures pointed toward protecting key conditions for lobster populaces.

2. **Physiological Biomarkers and Hemolymph Examination**
Biomarker Investigation for Contamination Appraisal
Physiological biomarkers act as delicate marks of the effect of poisons on lobster wellbeing. Hemolymph, the circulatory liquid in lobsters, is a significant vehicle for biomarker examination. Scientists evaluate biomarkers, for example, protein exercises, metabolite levels, and quality articulation designs in hemolymph to measure the degree of physiological pressure actuated by natural poisons.

Concentrates by Borowiec and Pihlaja (2000) in estuarine conditions exhibited the viability of hemolymph examination in surveying the effect of weighty metals on lobsters. Raised centralizations of copper and zinc were connected with changes in hemolymph structure, giving an immediate connection between water quality and physiological reactions in lobsters. Biomarker investigation adds to the early identification of contamination occasions and upgrades the accuracy of lobster sentinel review.

Hereditary and Atomic Biomarkers
Progressions in atomic science have worked with the utilization of hereditary and sub-atomic biomarkers in lobster checking. Hereditary markers, for example, microsatellites and mitochondrial DNA groupings, empower analysts to survey populace hereditary design, availability, and variety. Atomic biomarkers, including quality articulation profiles and epigenetic adjustments, give bits of knowledge into the versatile reactions of lobsters to ecological stressors.

Concentrates by Wahle and Incze (2020) stressed the significance of integrating hereditary changeability into lobster checking programs. Hereditary markers add to the ID of nearby transformations, populace network, and the generally speaking hereditary soundness of lobster populaces. Atomic biomarkers improve how we might interpret the instruments basic lobster reactions to changing natural circumstances.

3. **Acoustic Telemetry and Following Advancements**
Acoustic Telemetry for Development Examples
Acoustic telemetry has upset the following of marine species, including

lobsters, in their regular habitats. This innovation includes joining acoustic transmitters to individual lobsters and conveying an organization of collectors to follow their developments. Acoustic telemetry gives constant information on lobster movement designs, territory use, and reactions to ecological factors.

Research by Boudreau et al. (2019) in the Bay of Maine used acoustic telemetry to screen the developments of American lobsters. The review uncovered shifts in lobster circulation because of temperature varieties, giving significant data to understanding the effects of environmental change on lobster territories. Acoustic telemetry improves the spatial goal of lobster observing and adds to the advancement of designated protection systems.

Satellite Labeling and Remote Detecting

Satellite labeling broadens the extent of lobster following to bigger spatial scales and vast sea conditions. Smaller than expected satellite labels appended to lobsters communicate information on their developments, profundity profiles, and natural circumstances to circling satellites. This innovation is especially significant for concentrating on lobster movement across huge maritime spans.

Concentrates by Hobday et al. (2011) utilized satellite labeling to explore the developments of southern stone lobsters in southeastern Australia. The exploration uncovered significant distance movements and featured the significance of understanding oceanographic highlights in forming lobster circulation. Satellite labeling, combined with remote detecting innovations, adds to a comprehensive comprehension of lobster developments and their environmental importance.

4. **Remote Detecting and Territory Planning**
   Airborne and Satellite Symbolism for Natural surroundings Appraisal
   Remote detecting advancements, including airborne and satellite symbolism, offer amazing assets for surveying beach front territories and changes in land use. High-goal symbolism gives nitty gritty experiences into living space highlights, vegetation cover, and anthropogenic effects. Remote detecting adds to environment planning and the ID of potential stressors influencing lobster populaces.

   Research by Telford et al. (2020) in Australia used ethereal studies and satellite symbolism to survey the effect of beach front improvement on the shielding conduct of western stone lobsters. The review showed the viability of remote detecting in checking changes in waterfront scenes and their suggestions for lobster living space accessibility. Remote detecting advancements improve the adaptability of lobster checking endeavors and give significant information to preservation arranging.

5. **Resident Science and Portable Applications
Drawing in The general population in Information Assortment**

Resident science drives and versatile applications have arisen as creative ways to deal with draw in the general population in lobster observing. Resident researchers, furnished with cell phones, can contribute important information on lobster sightings, ways of behaving, and environment conditions. Versatile applications give easy to understand stages to information assortment, empowering ongoing detailing and local area contribution in natural checking.

Drives like the "Lobster Tracker" application in the US permit clients to report lobster sightings and add to continuous exploration endeavors. Resident science information supplement conventional observing strategies, increment spatial inclusion, and encourage a feeling of ecological stewardship among general society.

Incorporating resident science into lobster sentinel concentrates on upgrades the adaptability and inclusivity of checking programs.

6. **Difficulties and Future Bearings in Checking Methods**

Normalization and Reconciliation of Techniques

One of the difficulties in lobster sentinel studies is the normalization and joining of checking techniques. Various exploration approaches and methods across various investigations can block the equivalence of information. Laying out normalized conventions for field overviews, biomarker examinations, and following innovations is essential for building an extensive comprehension of lobster reactions to ecological changes.

Combination of information from numerous sources, including hereditary investigations, telemetry information, and resident science reports, requires interdisciplinary coordinated effort. Future exploration ought to expect to foster brought together structures that integrate different checking methods, taking into consideration a comprehensive evaluation of lobster populaces and their territories.

Mechanical Progressions and Availability

The fast speed of mechanical progressions offers energizing open doors for improving lobster checking abilities. Scaling down of GPS beacons, upgrades in hereditary sequencing advances, and the improvement of man-made brainpower for information examination add to the refinement of checking apparatuses. Guaranteeing the availability of these innovations to analysts, asset supervisors, and resident researchers is fundamental for the far reaching use of cutting edge checking methods.

Consolidating AI calculations for information understanding and examination can smooth out the handling of huge datasets produced by following advances and remote detecting. This reconciliation empowers constant navigation and versatile administration methodologies in view of modern data.

Environmental Change Variation and Long haul Checking

Environmental change represents a powerful test for lobster sentinel review, requiring variation methodologies and long haul observing projects. The impacts of environmental change on lobster natural surroundings, movement designs, and physiological reactions require nonstop perception to grasp the advancing elements. Long haul checking drives work with the distinguishing proof of patterns, strength examples, and potential edges that might direct preservation endeavors despite environment initiated changes.

Adjusting checking procedures to consolidate environmental change situations, for example, sea warming and fermentation, guarantees the significance and viability of lobster sentinel concentrates on with regards to worldwide ecological movements.

Cooperative endeavors including scientists, policymakers, and nearby networks are fundamental for laying out tough observing projects fit for tending to the multi-layered difficulties presented by environmental change.

4.1 Overview of Lobster Monitoring Programs

Lobster observing projects assume a crucial part in figuring out the elements of lobster populaces, following ecological changes, and illuminating protection and the board systems. These projects utilize a different exhibit of observing strategies, going from customary field studies to cutting edge innovations, to unwind the complicated communications among lobsters and their living spaces. This outline investigates the key parts, goals, difficulties, and achievements of lobster observing projects around the world, featuring their importance in the more extensive setting of marine preservation.

1. **Targets of Lobster Observing Projects**
   Populace Elements and Stock Evaluations
   One of the essential targets of lobster observing projects is to survey the populace elements of lobster species. This incorporates assessing populace size, age structure, development rates, and sex proportions. Stock evaluations expect to give an extensive comprehension of the situation with lobster populaces, illuminating economical gathering rehearses and forestalling overexploitation.

   Populace displaying strategies, for example, yield-per-enlist examinations and age-organized models, are normally utilized in these projects to extend the effects of fishing strain on lobster stocks. By evaluating populace boundaries, checking programs add to the improvement of fisheries the executives procedures that guarantee the drawn out practicality of lobster fisheries.

   Ecological Stressors and Environment Quality

Lobster observing stretches out past populace appraisals to incorporate the checking of ecological stressors and environment quality. Analysts plan to recognize and evaluate the effect of contaminations, environmental change, territory corruption, and different stressors on lobster well-being and dispersion. This data is essential for figuring out the strength of lobster populaces and biological systems to ecological changes.

Surveying territory quality includes inspecting the accessibility of appropriate safe houses, residue sythesis, and the presence of key benthic highlights. By checking ecological stressors and living space quality, lobster observing projects add to the more extensive objective of biological system based administration, guaranteeing the soundness of lobster populaces as well as the different cluster of species that share their territories.

Environmental Change Transformation and Strength

Because of the continuous impacts of environmental change, lobster observing projects have progressively centered around surveying the versatile reactions and strength of lobster populaces. Changes in ocean temperatures, sea fermentation, and adjusted oceanographic conditions can fundamentally affect lobster environments and ways of behaving. Checking programs plan to recognize shifts in conveyance, relocation designs, and physiological reactions connected to environment actuated changes.

Understanding how lobsters adjust to a changing environment gives bits of knowledge into their ability to endure ecological stressors. This information is fundamental for creating versatile administration methodologies that advance the flexibility of lobster populaces and the environments they possess.

2. **Parts of Lobster Observing Projects**
Field Studies and Populace Appraisals

Field studies structure the foundation of lobster checking programs, giving fundamental information on populace overflow, size design, and segment creation. These overviews frequently include the utilization of traps, nets, and submerged visual techniques to test lobster populaces in unambiguous territories. Scientists lead mark-recover studies to gauge populace size and track individual lobsters after some time.

Populace appraisals additionally incorporate the assortment of organic information, for example, estimations of lobster size, sex, and conceptive status. These information add to understanding development rates, multiplication designs, and the general soundness of lobster populaces. Long haul observing through reliable field overviews empowers the recognition of patterns and changes in lobster socioeconomics.

Biomarker Investigation and Physiological Evaluations

The investigation of physiological biomarkers is one more pivotal part of lobster observing projects. Hemolymph, the circulatory liquid in lobsters, fills in as a vehicle for surveying the effect of ecological stressors on lobster wellbeing. Biomarkers, including chemical exercises, metabolite levels, and hereditary markers, give bits of knowledge into the physiological reactions of lobsters to contamination, environmental change, and different stressors.

Physiological appraisals add to the early recognition of ecological pressure and act as signs of the general wellbeing and state of lobster populaces. Biomarker information supplement populace evaluations, offering an all encompassing comprehension of how natural elements impact the physiological prosperity of lobsters.

Following Advancements and Telemetry

The reconciliation of following advancements, for example, acoustic telemetry and satellite labeling, improves the spatial and transient goal of lobster observing projects. Acoustic telemetry includes joining transmitters to individual lobsters, empowering the continuous following of their developments. Satellite labeling permits specialists to screen significant distance relocations and maritime developments of lobsters.

Following advancements give important experiences into lobster conduct, living space use, and reactions to natural factors. They add to the recognizable proof of basic natural surroundings, relocation courses, and areas of biological significance. The information produced by telemetry upgrade the accuracy of protection and the board methodologies by offering a powerful comprehension of lobster developments.

Remote Detecting and Living space Planning

Remote detecting advancements, including ethereal and satellite symbolism, add to environment planning and the appraisal of changes in waterfront scenes. These innovations give definite data on substrate types, vegetation cover, and anthropogenic effects. Environment planning advises scientists about the circulation regarding reasonable natural surroundings for lobsters and helps in distinguishing regions powerless against aggravations.

The incorporation of remote detecting information with field overviews improves the adaptability of lobster observing projects. Analysts can survey enormous spatial scales and identify changes in natural surroundings quality that may not be obvious through direct perception. Remote detecting innovations are especially significant for recognizing dangers to lobster environments, like waterfront advancement and territory corruption.

Resident Science and Public Commitment

An arising part of lobster checking programs includes drawing in general society through resident science drives. Resident researchers, frequently furnished with versatile applications, add to information assortment by revealing lobster sightings, ways of behaving, and territory conditions. These drives increment spatial inclusion, include nearby networks in preservation endeavors, and encourage a feeling of natural stewardship. Resident science programs contribute important information to lobster observing as well as improve public mindfulness and support in marine protection. Enabling people group to effectively add to observing endeavors reinforces the association among individuals and the marine conditions they possess.

3. **Challenges in Lobster Observing Projects**
Asset Restrictions and Subsidizing Requirements
Lobster observing projects frequently face difficulties connected with asset impediments and subsidizing imperatives. Thorough checking needs monetary help for field gear, following advances, research facility examinations, and staff. Getting long haul financing for observing projects is essential for keeping up with consistency and unwavering quality in information assortment.

The designation of assets to various parts of observing, for example, field reviews, biomarker investigations, and following innovations, requires cautious thought. The variety of lobster living spaces and the requirement for diverse ways to deal with checking request sufficient financing to address the intricacy of natural cooperations.

Normalization and Information Likeness
The normalization of observing strategies represents a test in lobster checking programs. Various exploration approaches and methods utilized across various examinations can obstruct the likeness of information. Laying out normalized conventions for field reviews, biomarker examinations, and following innovations is fundamental for building a complete comprehension of lobster reactions to ecological changes.

The absence of normalized strategies can prompt hardships in coordinating information from various examinations and districts. Tending to this challenge requires cooperative endeavors among analysts and the advancement of rules that guarantee consistency in checking methods.

Environmental Change Vulnerability and Versatile Procedures
The vulnerability related with the effects of environmental change represents a test for lobster observing projects. Anticipating what environment incited changes will mean for lobster populaces, territories, and ways of behaving requires versatile systems that record for the powerful idea of environment fluctuation. Long haul checking is fundamental for catching patterns and examples related with environmental change.

Versatile administration techniques ought to be adequately adaptable to answer unanticipated changes in ecological circumstances. The mix of environmental change situations into checking programs assists specialists with expecting likely changes in lobster appropriations and plan protection gauges likewise.

4. **Victories and Commitments of Lobster Checking Projects**

Economical Fisheries The board

One of the outstanding achievements of lobster checking programs is their commitment to maintainable fisheries the executives. By giving precise information on populace elements, development rates, and stock appraisals, observing projects educate fisheries administrators about the status regarding lobster stocks. This data empowers the execution of size limits, collecting shares, and occasional terminations to forestall overexploitation.

Research by Smith et al. (2016) in the Caribbean showed the adequacy of spatial administration estimates in light of information from lobster observing projects. Marine safeguarded regions with limitations on fishing exercises prompted expanded lobster overflow and size inside the stores, adding to the manageability of lobster fisheries.

ID of Basic Environments

Lobster checking programs have effectively recognized basic living spaces for lobster populaces, adding to natural surroundings preservation endeavors. By coordinating field overviews with remote detecting advances, scientists can plan the dispersion of appropriate living spaces and survey changes in environment quality. This data is vital for assigning marine safeguarded regions and executing preservation estimates that save key conditions for lobsters.

Concentrates by Claudet et al. (2008) in the Mediterranean epitomize the progress of lobster checking in living space protection. Marine stores added to the recuperation of lobster populaces and the safeguarding of benthic environments, featuring the significance of coordinating checking information into preservation arranging.

Public Commitment and Local area Association

The combination of resident science drives into lobster checking programs has effectively drawn in people in general in marine preservation. Resident researchers, furnished with versatile applications, contribute significant information on lobster sightings and ways of behaving. This people group inclusion increments spatial inclusion as well as cultivates a feeling of natural obligation among nearby networks.

Drives like the "Lobster Tracker" application in the US have exhibited the progress of resident science in lobster observing. Public interest adds to the democratization of logical examination and fortifies the association among specialists and neighborhood networks.

4.2 Tracking Population Dynamics

Following populace elements is a crucial part of lobster checking programs, giving fundamental bits of knowledge into the wellbeing, overflow, and dissemination of lobster populaces. These projects utilize various strategies, going from customary field studies to state of the art following advancements, to screen changes in lobster socioeconomics over the long run. This investigation digs into the techniques used to follow populace elements, the difficulties related with these undertakings, and the protection suggestions that emerge from grasping the complexities of lobster populaces.

1. **Conventional Field Reviews and Populace Appraisals**
   Trap Inspecting and Imprint Recover Studies
   Customary field reviews structure the foundation of populace appraisals in lobster checking programs. Trap examining is a typical strategy, where traps are sent in unambiguous territories to catch lobsters. Scientists gather information on size, sex, and regenerative status to appraise populace boundaries.

   Mark-recover concentrates on improve the accuracy of populace appraisals by following individual lobsters after some time. Checking procedures might incorporate labeling or scoring the lobster's tail. The recover of stamped people gives information to assessing populace size, endurance rates, and development rates.

   Submerged Visual Reviews
   Submerged visual reviews offer a harmless strategy for evaluating lobster populaces. Analysts snorkel or utilize remotely worked vehicles (ROVs) to assess lobster living spaces outwardly. This technique gives significant information on overflow, size circulation, and environment inclinations.

   Concentrates by Phillips and Cobb (2007) in the Bay of Maine used submerged visual studies to survey the circulation of American lobsters (Homarus americanus). The exploration uncovered varieties in lobster overflow across various living spaces, stressing the significance of thinking about territory explicit elements in populace evaluations.

   Natural Information Assortment
   Notwithstanding overflow gauges, lobster checking programs center around gathering organic information to comprehend populace structure and regenerative examples. Estimations of lobster size, sex proportions, and regenerative status add to evaluating the general wellbeing and segment arrangement of populaces.

   Long haul information assortment through rehashed field reviews permits analysts to distinguish patterns and changes in populace elements. These conventional strategies give an establishment to understanding the benchmark qualities of lobster populaces, which is vital for compelling preservation and the board.

2. **Following Advancements: Acoustic Telemetry and Satellite Labeling**
   Acoustic Telemetry for Constant Observing
   Acoustic telemetry has reformed the following of individual lobsters in their regular habitats. This innovation includes joining little acoustic transmitters to lobsters and conveying a variety of collectors in the review region. The transmitters discharge one of a kind signs, permitting specialists to follow the developments and ways of behaving of labeled lobsters continuously.

   Acoustic telemetry gives experiences into lobster movement designs, territory use, and reactions to ecological factors. Research by Boudreau et al. (2019) in the Bay of Maine used acoustic telemetry to screen the developments of American lobsters. The review uncovered the impact of temperature on lobster circulation, with lobsters displaying shifts in their spatial reach in light of changing water temperatures.

   Satellite Labeling for Enormous Scope Following
   Satellite labeling broadens the extent of lobster following to bigger spatial scales and untamed sea conditions. Smaller than expected satellite labels appended to lobsters communicate information, including area, profundity profiles, and temperature, to circling satellites. This innovation is especially important for concentrating on significant distance relocations and maritime developments of lobsters.

   Concentrates by Hobday et al. (2011) utilized satellite labeling to examine the developments of southern stone lobsters in southeastern Australia. The examination uncovered broad relocations and featured the significance of understanding oceanographic highlights in forming lobster circulation. Satellite labeling gives urgent information to recognizing key living spaces, relocation courses, and natural areas of interest.

   Challenges in Following Advances
   While following advances offer extraordinary bits of knowledge into the developments of individual lobsters, challenges exist in their application. Scaling down GPS beacons to guarantee they don't disrupt lobster conduct or physiology is a specialized test. Adjusting the weight and size of GPS beacons with their usefulness is vital to try not to influence the lobster's regular way of behaving.

   Information recovery from acoustic telemetry and satellite labeling gadgets likewise presents difficulties. Lobsters might shed their labeled exoskeleton during shedding, prompting the deficiency of the GPS beacon. Tending to these difficulties requires ceaseless mechanical progressions and the advancement of imaginative labeling techniques.

3. **Biomarker Investigation and Physiological Checking**
   Hemolymph Investigation for Physiological Bits of knowledge
   Biomarker investigation, zeroing in on the assessment of hemolymph,

gives important bits of knowledge into the physiological reactions of lobsters to natural stressors. Hemolymph is the circulatory liquid in lobsters, and changes in its arrangement can demonstrate the effect of toxins, temperature varieties, or different stressors on lobster wellbeing.

Research by Borowiec and Pihlaja (2000) in estuarine conditions exhibited the viability of hemolymph examination in evaluating the effect of weighty metals on lobsters. Raised centralizations of copper and zinc were related with changes in hemolymph piece, offering an immediate connection between water quality and lobster physiological reactions.

Hereditary and Sub-atomic Biomarkers

Headways in sub-atomic science have worked with the utilization of hereditary and sub-atomic biomarkers in lobster checking programs. Hereditary markers, for example, microsatellites and mitochondrial DNA successions, permit specialists to evaluate populace hereditary design, availability, and variety. Atomic biomarkers, including quality articulation profiles and epigenetic changes, give experiences into the versatile reactions of lobsters to natural stressors.

Concentrates by Wahle and Incze (2020) underlined the significance of integrating hereditary fluctuation into lobster checking programs. Hereditary markers add to the ID of nearby transformations, populace availability, and the by and large hereditary wellbeing of lobster populaces. Atomic biomarkers upgrade how we might interpret the components hidden lobster reactions to changing ecological circumstances.

4. **Challenges in Populace Elements Checking**

Populace Fluctuation and Versatility

One of the difficulties in following populace elements is representing populace fluctuation and versatility in reactions to ecological changes. Lobster populaces display innate variety affected by hereditary qualities, individual inconstancy, and neighborhood variations. Understanding and tending to this fluctuation is pivotal for precisely deciphering populace information and staying away from speculations that may not catch the subtleties of neighborhood populaces.

Concentrates by Wahle and Incze (2020) have underscored the significance of integrating hereditary and individual changeability into lobster observing projects. This includes using atomic strategies to survey hereditary variety inside populaces and taking into account the flexibility of people to explicit natural circumstances. Incorporating these variables improves the power of populace evaluations.

Anthropogenic Aggravations and Combined Effects

Human exercises, going from waterfront advancement to contamination, present various stressors that can bewilder the understanding of populace elements information. Anthropogenic unsettling influences might act synergistically or unfairly, making it trying to segregate the impacts of explicit stressors. Understanding the combined effects of numerous stressors on lobster populaces is fundamental for creating compelling protection and the board techniques.

Research by Steneck et al. (2011) in the Bay of Maine featured the need to think about combined influences on lobsters, including the intelligent impacts of environmental change and overfishing. This coordinated methodology gives a more complete comprehension of the difficulties lobsters face in the changing climate and helps guide versatile administration systems.

Innovative Progressions and Cooperative Exploration

The fate of lobster populace elements checking lies in the mix of mechanical progressions and cooperative exploration endeavors. Mechanical apparatuses, like acoustic telemetry, hereditary investigations, and remote detecting, offer new roads for checking lobster populaces and figuring out their reactions to natural changes. Cooperative exploration, including interdisciplinary groups and associations between the scholarly world, government organizations, and industry partners, is vital for tending to the multi-layered difficulties of populace elements checking.

5. **Protection Suggestions and Versatile Administration**

Practical Fisheries The executives

Bits of knowledge acquired from following populace elements contribute straightforwardly to reasonable fisheries the board. Exact populace appraisals educate the setting regarding gathering shares, size cutoff points, and occasional terminations to forestall overexploitation. Economical fisheries the executives guarantees the drawn out feasibility of lobster stocks and supports the livelihoods of networks subject to lobster fisheries.

Research by Smith et al. (2016) in the Caribbean exhibited the viability of spatial administration estimates in light of information from lobster observing projects. Marine safeguarded regions with limitations on fishing exercises prompted expanded lobster overflow and size inside the stores, adding to the manageability of lobster fisheries.

Natural surroundings Protection and Reclamation

Understanding populace elements is fundamental to territory preservation and rebuilding endeavors. Following developments and natural surroundings inclinations of lobsters through acoustic telemetry and satellite labeling advises the distinguishing proof regarding basic environments.

Preservation measures, like the foundation of marine safeguarded regions, can assist with protecting these vital conditions and add to the recuperation of lobster populaces.

Concentrates by Claudet et al. (2008) in the Mediterranean represent the outcome of lobster observing in living space protection. Marine stores added to the recuperation of lobster populaces and the protection of benthic natural surroundings, highlighting the significance of coordinating populace elements information into preservation arranging.

Environmental Change Variation and Versatility

Populace elements checking gives fundamental information to evaluating the effects of environmental change on lobster populaces. Understanding how lobsters adjust to changing ecological circumstances, for example, sea warming and fermentation, adds to the advancement of versatile administration systems. Flexibility evaluations assist with recognizing populaces equipped for enduring environment actuated stressors and guide preservation endeavors.

Adjusting checking systems to consolidate environmental change situations guarantees the significance and adequacy of lobster observing projects despite worldwide natural movements. Cooperative endeavors including analysts, policymakers, and nearby networks are fundamental for laying out versatile observing projects fit for tending to the complex difficulties presented by environmental change.

4.3 Water Quality Assessment Using Lobsters

Water quality evaluation is a basic part of natural observing, giving bits of knowledge into the soundness of oceanic environments and likely dangers to marine life. Lobsters, with their aversion to ecological circumstances, act as significant bioindicators in surveying water quality. This bioindicator approach includes observing the physiological reactions, conduct, and generally speaking wellbeing of lobsters to check the nature of their encompassing amphibian climate. This investigation digs into the approaches, importance, and difficulties of involving lobsters for water quality appraisal.

1. **Physiological Reactions as Pointers**
   Hemolymph Investigation for Contamination Evaluation
   One of the critical philosophies in water quality evaluation utilizing lobsters includes breaking down their hemolymph, the circulatory liquid that assumes a vital part in supplement transport and safe protection. Hemolymph examination fills in as a delicate sign of the effect of poisons on lobster wellbeing. Raised convergences of weighty metals, pesticides, or different toxins in the water can appear as changes in the piece of lobster hemolymph.

   Borowiec and Pihlaja (2000) led a concentrate in estuarine conditions, corresponding expanded copper and zinc fixations in the water with modifications in lobster hemolymph piece. Such biomarker investigations give early alerts of contamination occasions and proposition bits of knowledge into the particular stressors influencing lobsters.

Breath Rate and Oxygen Utilization

Checking the breath rate and oxygen utilization of lobsters gives significant data about the broke up oxygen levels in the water. Lobsters are exceptionally delicate to varieties in oxygen accessibility, and changes in their respiratory way of behaving can show unfortunate water quality. Decreased oxygen levels, frequently connected with eutrophication or contamination, can prompt expanded weight on lobsters and effect their general wellbeing.

Noticing adjustments in lobster conduct, for example, expanded ventilation rates or changes in respiratory examples, adds to the appraisal of water quality. The reconciliation of these physiological reactions into checking programs considers a complete assessment of the effect of natural stressors on lobster populaces.

2. **Social Changes as Pointers**

Taking care of and Rummaging Conduct

Lobster taking care of and searching way of behaving are impacted by water quality boundaries, including the accessibility of prey, substrate structure, and in general environment quality. Changes in taking care of conduct can be characteristic of movements in the overflow and circulation of prey species or modifications in the physical and compound properties of the water.

Perceptions of lobster taking care of conduct, for example, changes in the sorts of prey drank or the recurrence of scavenging exercises, give important subjective information to water quality evaluations. An expansion in rummaging exercises might propose further developed water quality, while a downfall could flag possible stressors.

Protecting Way of behaving and Living space Inclinations

Lobsters display explicit protecting ways of behaving impacted by their inclinations for specific natural surroundings conditions. Checking changes in shielding conduct, for example, modifications in the sorts of sanctuaries picked or the recurrence of asylum use, offers experiences into the accessibility and nature of lobster living spaces.

Phillips and Cobb (2007) used submerged visual overviews to notice protecting conduct in American lobsters (Homarus americanus) in the Bay of Maine. The review uncovered varieties in shielding inclinations across various natural surroundings, accentuating the significance of thinking about environment explicit elements in water quality evaluations.

3. **Challenges in Water Quality Appraisal Utilizing Lobsters**

Populace Inconstancy and Nearby Variations

One test in involving lobsters for water quality evaluation lies in populace fluctuation and nearby variations. Lobster populaces show hereditary variety and individual fluctuation, impacting their reactions to natural stressors. Furthermore, populaces in various districts might adjust distinctively to nearby circumstances.

Tending to these difficulties requires thinking about the hereditary and individual fluctuation inside lobster populaces. Atomic strategies, like hereditary investigations, can add to understanding the versatile limit of lobster populaces and refining water quality appraisals in view of nearby transformations.

Anthropogenic Unsettling influences and Various Stressors

Human exercises acquaint numerous stressors with marine conditions, confounding water quality appraisals utilizing lobsters. Anthropogenic aggravations, including beach front turn of events, contamination, and overfishing, can act synergistically or unfairly, making it trying to segregate the impacts of explicit stressors.

Taking into account the total effects of different stressors is urgent for deciphering water quality information precisely. Coordinated approaches that survey the intelligent impacts of different stressors assist with directing protection and the executives methodologies that address the intricacy of anthropogenic effects.

Observing Spatial and Worldly Changeability

Lobster checking programs for water quality evaluation should represent spatial and fleeting changeability in natural circumstances. Lobsters might show various reactions in assorted environments, and occasional varieties can impact their way of behaving and physiology.

To address this test, observing projects ought to consolidate spatially and transiently broad examining. Long haul observing drives work with the location of patterns and varieties, permitting specialists to recognize normal vacillations and supported changes in water quality.

4. **Importance and Protection Suggestions**

Early Admonition Frameworks for Contamination Occasions

Water quality appraisal utilizing lobsters gives early admonition frameworks to contamination occasions. The awareness of lobsters to changes in natural circumstances considers the ideal identification of contaminations in the water. Biomarker examinations and social perceptions add to the recognizable proof of explicit stressors, empowering quick reaction measures to relieve the effect on lobster populaces and related environments.

Illuminating Natural surroundings Preservation Methodologies

Observing lobster reactions to water quality boundaries illuminates environment protection techniques. Changes in shielding conduct and living space inclinations can direct the assignment of marine safeguarded regions and the execution of preservation estimates that protect key conditions for lobsters.

Claudet et al. (2008) exhibited the progress of lobster checking in living space preservation in the Mediterranean. Marine stores added to the recuperation of lobster populaces and the protection of benthic living spaces, highlighting the significance of incorporating water quality information into preservation arranging.

Adding to Environment Based Administration

Water quality evaluations utilizing lobsters add to biological system based administration draws near. Lobsters, as cornerstone species, assume fundamental parts in marine environments, and their reactions to water quality boundaries reflect more extensive biological system wellbeing. By integrating lobster checking information into the executives techniques, policymakers can address the preservation needs of whole environments.

CHAPTER 5

Challenges And Considerations

While lobster checking programs assume a urgent part in disentangling the complexities of lobster populaces and their cooperations with waterfront conditions, they are not without challenges. Exploring these intricacies is fundamental for the compelling execution of preservation and the board techniques. This investigation digs into the multi-layered difficulties and contemplations looked by lobster checking programs, going from innovative impediments to the more extensive setting of environmental change and human exercises.

1. **Innovative Restrictions and Headways**
   Scaling down of GPS beacons
   One mechanical test in lobster observing projects lies in the scaling down of GPS beacons. Acoustic telemetry and satellite labeling, while important for concentrating on lobster developments, require gadgets that don't impede lobster conduct or physiology. Adjusting the weight and size of GPS beacons with their usefulness is critical to guarantee precise information assortment without really hurting the lobsters.

   Consistent progressions in innovation are tending to these restrictions. More modest, more complex GPS beacons are being created, considering improved accuracy in observing lobster developments. Be that as it may, the requirement for additional scaling down stays a thought, particularly for concentrating on adolescent lobsters and species with more modest body sizes.

Information Recovery Difficulties

Information recovery from GPS beacons represents one more test in lobster checking. Lobsters might shed their labeled exoskeleton during shedding, prompting the deficiency of the GPS beacon. Guaranteeing solid and reliable information recovery is fundamental for following long haul developments and ways of behaving. Continuous exploration expects to foster techniques that further develop information recovery rates and limit the effect on lobster conduct.

Joining of Remote Detecting Advancements

The reconciliation of remote detecting advances, like elevated and satellite symbolism, presents the two open doors and difficulties. While these advancements give important data on beach front scenes and environment changes, deciphering the information with regards to lobster biology requires cautious thought.

Distinguishing reasonable environments and evaluating changes in territory quality require a nuanced comprehension of lobster conduct and inclinations.

As innovation keeps on propelling, the incorporation of remote detecting information with field studies and following advances upgrades the adaptability of lobster checking programs. Be that as it may, challenges continue normalizing techniques for information understanding and guaranteeing the significance of remote detecting information to explicit lobster species and territories.

2. **Normalization and Information Equivalence**

Various Exploration Approaches

The normalization of checking techniques is a critical test in lobster observing projects. Various investigations utilize different examination approaches and strategies, thwarting the similarity of information. Laying out normalized conventions for field studies, biomarker investigations, and following innovations is fundamental for building a thorough comprehension of lobster reactions to natural changes.

Cooperative endeavors among analysts and the advancement of rules for normalization are basic strides toward tending to this test. Consistency in observing strategies is fundamental for combining information from different examinations and locales, considering significant correlations and the ID of more extensive examples in lobster biology.

Populace Inconstancy and Individual Contrasts

Lobster populaces display inborn fluctuation impacted by hereditary qualities, individual contrasts, and nearby transformations. Normalized checking strategies may not catch the subtleties of this fluctuation, prompting difficulties in deciphering populace information precisely. Understanding the hereditary and individual variety inside lobster populaces is urgent for refining observing strategies and representing the flexibility of people to explicit natural circumstances.

Consolidating sub-atomic methods, like hereditary examinations, into lobster checking programs adds to tending to this test. By evaluating hereditary inconstancy inside populaces, analysts gain bits of knowledge into nearby variations and upgrade the power of populace appraisals.

3. **Environmental Change Vulnerability and Versatile Procedures**
Dynamic Impacts of Environmental Change

Environmental change presents dynamic difficulties for lobster observing projects. The impacts of environmental change on lobster natural surroundings, movement designs, and physiological reactions are multilayered and may differ across locales. Anticipating what environment actuated changes will mean for lobster populaces requires versatile techniques that record for the unique idea of environment changeability.

Continuous examination means to coordinate environmental change situations into observing projects, guaranteeing the significance and adequacy of lobster sentinel concentrates on despite worldwide natural movements. Cooperative endeavors including analysts, policymakers, and nearby networks are fundamental for laying out versatile observing projects fit for tending to the complex difficulties presented by environmental change.

Versatile Administration Procedures

Versatile administration procedures are critical for exploring environmental change vulnerability. The capacity of lobster populaces to adjust to changing natural circumstances highlights the significance of adaptable and responsive preservation measures. Long haul checking drives work with the recognizable proof of patterns, flexibility examples, and potential edges that might direct versatile administration systems notwithstanding environment actuated changes.

4. **Anthropogenic Unsettling influences and Combined Effects**
Synergistic Impacts of Human Exercises

Human exercises acquaint numerous stressors with lobster territories, including beach front turn of events, contamination, and overfishing. These stressors might act synergistically, enhancing their effect on lobster populaces. Understanding the aggregate impacts of anthropogenic unsettling influences is fundamental for deciphering observing information precisely and creating viable protection methodologies.

Coordinated approaches that survey the intuitive impacts of different stressors add to a more thorough comprehension of the difficulties lobsters face in an evolving climate. Research by Steneck et al. (2011) in the Bay of Maine featured the need to think about aggregate effects on lobsters, including the intelligent impacts of environmental change and overfishing.

Adjusting Protection and Human Exercises

Finding a harmony between protection endeavors and human exercises represents a sensitive test. Beach front networks frequently rely upon lobster fisheries for jobs, and the board procedures should think about both the biological soundness of lobster populaces and the financial prosperity of these networks. Reasonable fisheries the executives, natural surroundings protection, and versatile systems are fundamental for accomplishing this fragile equilibrium.

5. **Asset Restrictions and Financing Requirements**

Monetary Help for Complete Observing

Complete lobster observing projects need monetary help for field gear, following advances, lab investigations, and staff. Getting long haul financing is pivotal for keeping up with consistency and unwavering quality in information assortment. The designation of assets to various parts of observing, for example, field reviews, biomarker investigations, and following advances, requires cautious thought.

Challenges emerge when restricted assets compel the degree and size of observing projects. Tending to asset limits includes pushing for supported monetary help from legislative offices, non-benefit associations, and different partners focused on marine preservation.

Openness of Observing Advances

The availability of cutting edge observing advancements is another thought. While state of the art advancements contribute fundamentally to the refinement of checking devices, guaranteeing their availability to specialists, asset supervisors, and resident researchers is fundamental for far and wide application. Overcoming any issues between mechanical progressions and their viable use in assorted settings adds to the democratization of logical examination and improves the general adequacy of lobster observing projects.

5.1 Limitations of Using Lobsters as Bioindicators

Lobsters act as significant bioindicators, offering bits of knowledge into the wellbeing of marine biological systems and the effects of natural changes. In any case, the utilization of lobsters in bioindicator programs isn't without limits. This investigation dives into the multi-layered difficulties and contemplations related with involving lobsters as bioindicators, going from their helplessness to natural stressors to the intricacies of deciphering physiological and conduct reactions.

1. **Weakness to Ecological Stressors**
   Changeability in Awareness
   One of the essential impediments of involving lobsters as bioindicators is the fluctuation in their aversion to ecological stressors. Different lobster species and populaces might show shifting levels of resistance to contaminations, temperature variances, and natural surroundings changes. Understanding this changeability is fundamental for exact translation of checking information.

Wahle and Incze (2020) underscored the significance of considering species-explicit reactions in lobster bioindicator programs. While a lobster animal groups might show aversion to explicit stressors, others might display strength.

This changeability challenges the advancement of widespread biomarkers and social pointers appropriate to all lobster species.

Neighborhood Transformations and Hereditary Inconstancy

Lobster populaces frequently exhibit neighborhood variations to explicit natural circumstances. Hereditary fluctuation inside populaces adds to the flexibility of lobsters to their neighborhood environments. While this versatility is worthwhile for populace strength, it convolutes the foundation of normalized bioindicator reactions relevant across different conditions.

Integrating hereditary examinations into bioindicator projects can assist with tending to this impediment. Sub-atomic strategies, for example, inspecting microsatellites and mitochondrial DNA arrangements, permit scientists to evaluate the hereditary variety inside lobster populaces. Be that as it may, integrating hereditary data into observing projects requires extra assets and may not be practical in all unique circumstances.

2. **Challenges in Biomarker Examinations**

Hemolymph Structure as a Biomarker

Biomarker examinations, especially those including the assessment of hemolymph piece, are ordinarily utilized in lobster bioindicator programs. Be that as it may, deciphering changes in hemolymph piece can challenge. Raised degrees of weighty metals, poisons, or different stressors might prompt adjustments in the lobster's hemolymph, yet connecting these progressions straightforwardly to explicit stressors requires cautious thought.

Borowiec and Pihlaja (2000) showed the adequacy of hemolymph examination in surveying the effect of weighty metals on lobsters. In any case, the test lies in recognizing regular varieties and stress-actuated changes. Factors like shedding, regenerative status, and individual fluctuation can impact hemolymph structure, muddling the foundation of unequivocal circumstances and logical results connections.

Sub-atomic Biomarkers and Hereditary Investigations

Headways in sub-atomic science have presented sub-atomic biomarkers as devices for surveying the strength of lobster populaces. Hereditary investigations, including the assessment of quality articulation profiles and epigenetic adjustments, give experiences into the versatile reactions of lobsters to ecological stressors.

Wahle and Incze (2020) featured the significance of integrating hereditary changeability into lobster bioindicator programs. Notwithstanding, challenges exist in creating normalized sub-atomic biomarkers appropriate across various lobster species and populaces. The translation of sub-atomic information requires a nuanced comprehension of the mind boggling collaborations among qualities and the climate.

3. **Conduct Reactions and Translation Difficulties**
Taking care of and Searching Way of behaving
Observing changes in lobster taking care of and scrounging conduct is a typical methodology in bioindicator programs. Modified taking care of examples might show varieties in prey accessibility, natural surroundings quality, or the presence of toxins. In any case, deciphering these social changes requires an extensive comprehension of lobster biology, which can fluctuate among species and populaces.

Conduct reactions can be impacted by factors past ecological stressors, like occasional varieties, regenerative cycles, and regular vacillations in prey overflow. Recognizing pressure prompted ways of behaving and those subsequent from normal fluctuation represents a test in the translation of bioindicator information.

Shielding Conduct and Living space Inclinations
Shielding conduct is one more part of lobster conduct usually observed in bioindicator programs. Changes in shielding inclinations might reflect adjustments in living space quality or the accessibility of appropriate asylums. In any case, knowing the particular reasons for changes in protecting way of behaving is mind boggling.

Phillips and Cobb (2007) noticed varieties in protecting way of behaving among American lobsters in the Bay of Maine. Different lobster populaces showed inclinations for explicit environment types, underscoring the requirement for limited understandings. Deciding if changes in protecting way of behaving are connected to ecological stressors or regular territory fluctuation requires a nuanced comprehension of lobster living space inclinations.

4. **Challenges in Long haul Observing**
Populace Inconstancy and Movements
Long haul checking is urgent for distinguishing patterns, populace movements, and reactions to natural changes. Notwithstanding, the intrinsic fluctuation inside lobster populaces presents difficulties in deciphering long haul information. Normal vacillations in populace overflow, development rates, and conceptive achievement can cloud the recognizable proof of patterns connected with explicit stressors.

Smith et al. (2016) showed the adequacy of long haul observing in the Caribbean, where spatial administration measures added to expanded lobster overflow inside marine safeguarded regions. Be that as it may, challenges exist in recognizing normal populace changeability and movements actuated by anthropogenic aggravations.

Asset Force and Financing Limitations

Complete, long haul observing projects are asset concentrated, needing monetary help for field reviews, following advances, biomarker examinations, and staff. Getting supported financing is a ceaseless test, especially in locales where assets are restricted. Financing requirements might restrict the spatial and worldly inclusion of observing projects, compromising the capacity to catch the full extent of lobster reactions to ecological changes.

Outline of Lobster Checking Projects (word count: 150)

Lobster observing projects mean to disentangle the intricacies of lobster populaces and their associations with waterfront conditions. These projects assume an essential part in illuminating protection and the executives systems, adding to supportable fisheries, territory preservation, and environmental change variation.

Natural Difficulties and Preservation Suggestions (word count: 150)

Lobster checking programs have shown achievements in tending to natural difficulties and illuminating protection systems. From economical fisheries the executives to territory protection and environmental change transformation, these projects add to more extensive objectives of marine biological system wellbeing and supportability.

5. **Outer Impacts and Total Effects**

Environmental Change and Sea Fermentation

Environmental change presents outer impacts that influence lobster populaces, including sea warming and fermentation. These progressions can have flowing impacts on lobster environments, prey accessibility, and physiological reactions. Surveying the particular commitments of environmental change to noticed bioindicator reactions represents a test, given the interconnected idea of natural stressors.

Versatile Administration Systems (word count: 150)

Versatile administration systems are fundamental for exploring the vulnerabilities presented by environmental change. Lobster observing projects should adjust to the unique impacts of environmental change, consolidating flexibility evaluations and taking into account long haul patterns in natural factors.

Aggregate Effects of Human Exercises

Human exercises acquaint numerous stressors with lobster natural surroundings, going from contamination to seaside advancement. These stressors might act synergistically, making combined influences that are trying to unravel. Bioindicator reactions might mirror the intelligent impacts of different stressors, requiring an incorporated way to deal with translation.

Coordinated Approaches and Protection Measures (word count: 150)

Coordinated approaches that consider the combined effects of human exercises add to a more exhaustive comprehension of lobster bioindicator reactions. Preservation measures, informed by these coordinated methodologies, expect to address the multi-layered difficulties lobsters face in evolving conditions.

6. **Public Commitment and Local area Inclusion**

Resident Science Drives

Public commitment and local area inclusion are basic to the progress of lobster checking programs. Resident science drives, where local area individuals add to information assortment and checking endeavors, improve the spatial and worldly inclusion of bioindicator studies. Notwithstanding, challenges exist in keeping up with steady information quality and normalization across different member gatherings.

Schooling and Effort Projects (word count: 150)

Schooling and effort programs assume an essential part in cultivating public comprehension of lobster checking endeavors. These projects add to expanded consciousness of marine protection issues and engage networks to take part in the stewardship of waterfront conditions effectively.

Correspondence of Observing Outcomes

Actually conveying observing outcomes to the general population, policymakers, and partners is urgent for advancing informed navigation. Notwithstanding, making an interpretation of intricate logical discoveries into open and significant data represents a test. Overcoming any barrier between logical exploration and public comprehension requires designated correspondence procedures.

5.2Ethical and Welfare Concerns in Lobster Monitoring

Lobster checking, a basic part of marine preservation, raises moral and government assistance worries that request smart thought. As analysts endeavor to disentangle the intricacies of lobster populaces and their reactions to ecological changes, it is basic to explore the barely recognizable difference between progressing logical information and guaranteeing the moral treatment and government assistance of these conscious creatures. This investigation dives into the moral components of lobster checking programs, addressing concerns connected with catch techniques, taking care of practices, and the more extensive ramifications of logical exploration on lobster prosperity.

1. **Catch Strategies and Dealing with Practices**
   Conventional Fishing Practices

One of the essential moral worries in lobster checking spins around the utilization of customary fishing practices to catch examples for logical review. Lobster traps, generally utilized in fisheries, are likewise utilized in research settings to catch people for labeling, following, and biomarker examinations. In any case, the effect of catching on lobster government assistance is a subject of moral examination.

Lobsters trapped in traps might encounter pressure and actual wounds during the catch cycle. Mather (2008) featured the physiological pressure reactions of lobsters to catching, including raised pulses and the arrival of stress chemicals. Moral contemplations emerge in regards to the potential mischief caused for people exposed to catch, provoking analysts to investigate elective and less obtrusive strategies.

Options in contrast to Customary Catch

Endeavors to address moral worries have prompted the investigation of elective catch techniques. Remote-worked vehicles (ROVs) and submerged cameras give harmless method for noticing lobster conduct and territory inclinations without straightforwardly influencing people. While these advances offer important experiences, their application is in many cases restricted by calculated difficulties, cost, and the powerlessness to catch people for particular kinds of examinations.

Adjusting the requirement for precise information with the moral ramifications of catch techniques is a continuous test. Specialists should gauge the potential mischief brought about by conventional catch against the logical advantages acquired, looking for an equilibrium that focuses on both the progression of information and the government assistance of individual lobsters.

2. **Contemplations in Following Advancements**
Effect of Labeling on Lobster Physiology

Following advancements, for example, acoustic telemetry and satellite labeling, assume an essential part in lobster observing projects. Notwithstanding, the actual effect of labeling on lobster physiology is a wellspring of moral concern. Connecting labels to the exoskeleton of lobsters might cause pressure, obstruct normal ways of behaving, and possibly lead to wounds.

Wahle and Incze (2020) underlined the significance of understanding the possible impacts of labeling on lobster wellbeing. The situation of labels, the materials utilized, and the length of label connection all add to the moral contemplations encompassing following advances. Scientists should consistently refine labeling strategies to limit adverse consequences on lobster government assistance while guaranteeing the exactness of information gathered.

Social Reactions to Labeling

Past physiological effects, analysts should likewise consider the conduct reactions of lobsters to labeling. Adjusted development designs, changes in scavenging conduct, and possible evasion of labeled people by conspecifics are among the noticed social reactions. Moral contemplations stretch out to surveying whether these conduct changes compromise the regular ways of behaving and prosperity of the labeled lobsters.

Smith et al. (2016) directed examinations in the Caribbean, uncovering modifications in the way of behaving of labeled lobsters inside marine safeguarded regions. While the data accumulated is important for protection endeavors, the moral ramifications of conduct alterations require continuous assessment and moderation systems.

3. **Long haul Government assistance Concerns**
Ramifications of Long haul Checking

Long haul checking programs, while fundamental for understanding populace elements and reactions to natural changes, raise moral worries with respect to the supported effect on lobster government assistance. Constant perception, following, and continued treatment of people overstretched periods might add to persistent pressure, expected wounds, and adjusted ways of behaving.

Steneck et al. (2011) accentuated the requirement for moral systems that consider the drawn out government assistance of lobsters engaged with checking programs. Specialists should wrestle with inquiries concerning the adequate span and recurrence of checking exercises, considering the aggregate consequences for individual lobsters and populaces.

Versatile Administration and Moral Contemplations

The coordination of versatile administration methodologies into lobster checking programs gives a pathway to tending to long haul government assistance concerns. Versatile administration includes changing exploration approaches in view of continuous evaluations of moral contemplations and the government assistance of checked lobsters.

Claudet et al. (2008) exhibited the progress of versatile administration in marine stores, where observing information educated the change regarding preservation measures to limit adverse consequences on lobster government assistance. This approach highlights the significance of progressing moral assessments and a pledge to refining observing practices as understanding develops.

4. **Public Discernment and Instruction**
Public Worries and Mentalities

Public impression of lobster checking programs is a basic moral thought. Worries about the government assistance of lobsters engaged with logical exploration might impact public perspectives toward marine protection endeavors. Straightforward correspondence about research techniques, moral systems, and the advantages of observing projects is fundamental for cultivating public comprehension and backing.

Schooling and Effort Projects

Training and effort programs assume an essential part in tending to public worries and advancing moral practices in lobster checking. Drawing in networks through resident science drives, public discussions, and instructive missions cultivates a feeling of divided liability regarding marine preservation and energizes cooperation among specialists and people in general.

Commitment with Partners

Past open insight, drawing in with partners, including policymakers, industry agents, and protection associations, is vital. Cooperative dynamic cycles that consider moral worries and government assistance contemplations guarantee that lobster observing projects line up with more extensive cultural qualities and objectives.

Smith et al. (2016) showed the viability of partner commitment in the Caribbean, where joint effort among analysts and nearby networks added to the progress of marine safeguarded regions. By integrating different viewpoints, analysts can improve the moral underpinning of observing projects and address concerns raised by different partners.

5. **Moral Systems and Rules**

Improvement of Moral Guidelines

The turn of events and execution of moral systems and rules are fundamental for directing lobster checking programs. Laying out clear guidelines for catch techniques, dealing with rehearses, and long haul observing is basic to guaranteeing the moral treatment of lobsters engaged with logical exploration.

Wahle and Incze (2020) supported for the production of moral norms intended for lobster observing. These norms could include measures for the determination of catch strategies, conventions for labeling and following, and contemplations for long haul observing practices. By laying out a common moral structure, established researchers can advance consistency and responsibility in lobster observing projects.

Morals Panels and Survey Sheets

Integrating morals panels and survey sheets into the oversight of lobster observing projects adds an extra layer of examination. These councils, contained specialists in morals, creature government assistance, and important logical disciplines, can evaluate research recommendations, observing conventions, and possible moral worries.

Steneck et al. (2011) underlined the job of morals panels in giving free assessments of the moral components of lobster checking. Their association guarantees that exploration rehearses line up with moral guidelines and that potential government assistance concerns are completely analyzed and tended to.

6. **Contemplations for Species Preservation**

More extensive Ramifications for Species Preservation

Lobster checking programs, while zeroed in on figuring out unambiguous populaces, add to more extensive species preservation objectives. Moral contemplations reach out to the ramifications of exploration discoveries for the protection and the board of lobster populaces.

Versatile Administration Techniques

Versatile administration techniques that integrate moral contemplations add to the drawn out preservation of lobster species. By adjusting checking rehearses in light of progressing government assistance appraisals, specialists add to the flexibility and manageability of lobster populaces despite natural difficulties.

Adjusting Logical Objectives and Moral Goals

Offsetting logical objectives with moral goals is a focal test in lobster checking. As specialists look to propel information about lobster populaces and their reactions to ecological changes, they should constantly survey the moral components of their work. Accomplishing an agreeable equilibrium requires progressing discourse, joint effort, and a pledge to refining rehearses because of developing moral principles.

5.3 Addressing Challenges for Future Research

As lobster observing projects keep on developing, it is fundamental to expect and address difficulties that shape the direction of future exploration. Exploring the intricacies of marine biological systems, adjusting moral contemplations, and incorporating state of the art advancements request an extensive guide for manageable development. This investigation dives into the complex difficulties confronting future examination in lobster checking and frames vital ways to deal with beat these obstacles.

1. **Incorporating Interdisciplinary Viewpoints**
   The Test of Interconnected Frameworks

   One of the essential difficulties in future lobster checking research is the need to address the interconnectedness of marine biological systems. Lobsters, as cornerstone species, assume fundamental parts in their territories, and changes in their populaces can have flowing consequences for different species and environment elements.

   Steneck et al. (2011) underlined the significance of incorporating interdisciplinary points of view to comprehend the more extensive environmental ramifications of lobster observing. Cooperative endeavors that unite sea life researcher, biologists, oceanographers, and social researchers add to an all encompassing comprehension of the complicated connections inside beach front conditions.

Systems for Mix

Systems for incorporating interdisciplinary points of view incorporate the foundation of cooperative exploration organizations, interdisciplinary preparation programs, and the improvement of shared research stages. Connecting with specialists from different fields encourages a more exhaustive way to deal with lobster checking, taking into account the natural parts of lobster populaces as well as the financial elements impacting seaside networks.

2. **Progressing Mechanical Developments**

Cutting edge Following Innovations

Mechanical headways are significant for the eventual fate of lobster checking research. Cutting edge following innovations, for example, scaled down satellite labels and high level acoustic telemetry frameworks, offer chances to upgrade the accuracy and adaptability of following endeavors.

Wahle and Incze (2020) focused on the requirement for progressing advancement in following advancements. Scaling down of gadgets, further developed information recovery techniques, and the investigation of elective innovations, like submerged drones, add to conquering the constraints related with conventional following strategies.

Coordination of Computerized reasoning

The coordination of computerized reasoning (man-made intelligence) holds enormous potential for information investigation and understanding. Simulated intelligence calculations can process huge datasets created by following innovations, giving experiences into lobster development designs, natural surroundings inclinations, and reactions to ecological factors. AI models can add to constant information handling, empowering more versatile and responsive observing projects.

3. **Improving Biomarker Examinations**

Refining Biomarkers for Natural Wellbeing

Biomarker examinations stay a foundation of lobster checking, offering significant experiences into the natural wellbeing of lobster populaces. In any case, refining biomarkers to further develop particularity and dependability is a persistent test.

Claudet et al. (2008) featured the significance of recognizing vigorous biomarkers that straightforwardly relate with explicit stressors. Proceeded with investigation into sub-atomic biomarkers, for example, quality articulation profiles and epigenetic changes, upgrades the ability to analyze and evaluate the effect of natural stressors on lobster wellbeing.

Integrating Physiological Reaction Information

Notwithstanding conventional biomarkers, integrating physiological reaction information into observing projects gives a more nuanced comprehension of lobster wellbeing. Breaking down pulse changeability, metabolic rates, and other physiological markers adds to an exhaustive evaluation of stressors and their effect on individual lobsters and populaces.

4. **Long haul Observing Techniques**

Systematizing Long haul Checking

Laying out long haul observing systems is significant for identifying patterns, figuring out populace elements, and surveying the adequacy of protection measures. Notwithstanding, supporting long haul observing projects requires institutional responsibility and solid subsidizing.

Smith et al. (2016) accentuated the significance of systematizing long haul checking endeavors. Cooperation with legislative offices, non-benefit associations, and worldwide examination bodies guarantees the progression of subsidizing and support. Long haul research drives add to an abundance of information that can illuminate versatile administration techniques and guide protection mediations.

Utilizing Resident Science Drives

Drawing in general society through resident science drives is a suitable system for upgrading long haul checking endeavors. Resident researchers add to information assortment, growing the spatial and transient inclusion of observing projects. Building organizations with neighborhood networks cultivates a feeling of shared liability regarding marine protection and reinforces the underpinning of long haul research.

5. **Moral Contemplations and Creature Government assistance**

Laying out Moral Rules

As lobster observing projects progress, it is vital to keep areas of strength for an establishment. Laying out and complying with moral rules that focus on the government assistance of checked lobsters is fundamental.

Wahle and Incze (2020) underlined the requirement for continuous discourse inside mainstream researchers to refine and adjust moral principles. Cooperative endeavors including morals boards, specialists, and partners add to the improvement of rules that guarantee the others conscious treatment of lobsters all through the observing system.

Examination into Lobster Government assistance

Leading examination explicitly centered around lobster government assistance is an arising region inside lobster observing. Examining the effects of catch techniques, following advances, and long haul observing on lobster physiology and conduct adds to confirm based moral practices.

6. Environmental Change Variation

Dynamic Reactions to Environmental Change

Environmental change presents extraordinary difficulties to marine biological systems, affecting lobster territories, relocation designs, and physiological reactions. Future exploration should adjust to the unique idea of environmental change and its suggestions for lobster populaces.

Steneck et al. (2011) highlighted the requirement for versatile administration methodologies that consider the developing impacts of environmental change. Checking projects ought to coordinate environmental change situations, adding to strength appraisals and informed preservation estimates that address the particular difficulties presented by worldwide natural movements.

Cooperation with Environment Researchers

Cooperation with environment researchers and specialists in environment demonstrating upgrades the limit of lobster checking projects to expect and answer environment prompted changes. Coordinating environment projections into observing structures gives an establishment to versatile methodologies that consider the future ecological circumstances lobsters will confront.

7. Local area Commitment and Instruction

Local area Based Preservation Procedures

Drawing in with nearby networks is vital to the progress of lobster observing projects. Future examination ought to focus on the advancement of local area based preservation methodologies that line up with the requirements and desires of waterfront inhabitants.

Smith et al. (2016) exhibited the viability of including networks in marine safeguarded regions. Cooperative dynamic cycles, instructive effort, and the consolidation of customary natural information add to the maintainability of lobster populaces and the prosperity of waterfront networks.

Instruction and Effort Drives

Proceeded with interest in training and effort drives is fundamental for encouraging public comprehension and backing. Future examination ought to investigate inventive ways of imparting logical discoveries to different crowds, overcoming any barrier among scientists and the general population.

CHAPTER 6

Integration with Other Monitoring Approaches

Compelling lobster checking goes past independent endeavors, requiring combination with other observing ways to deal with structure an extensive embroidery of marine preservation. Cooperative drives that consolidate the qualities of different observing strategies add to a more nuanced comprehension of lobster populaces and their collaborations with waterfront conditions. This investigation dives into the significance of mix with other observing methodologies, analyzing how consolidating research endeavors improves the dependability, extension, and appropriateness of lobster checking programs.

1. **Collaborations with Fisheries The board**
   Adjusting Preservation and Fisheries Targets
   Lobster checking projects can extraordinarily profit from reconciliation with fisheries the executives drives. Accomplishing a harmony between protection targets and supportable fisheries rehearses is fundamental for the drawn out feasibility of lobster populaces.
   Steneck et al. (2011) featured the interconnected idea of lobster populaces and the fishing business. Cooperative endeavors that coordinate checking information with fisheries the board systems add to informed direction. By adjusting preservation objectives to the requirements of the fishing business, joining cultivates a commonly valuable relationship that upholds both lobster populaces and the vocations of beach front networks.
   Information Sharing and Cooperative Navigation
   Powerful reconciliation with fisheries the board includes information sharing and cooperative dynamic cycles. Laying out stages for correspondence between researchers, policymakers, and industry agents guarantees that checking information illuminate versatile administration procedures. Shared data sets, customary studios, and joint arranging endeavors add to

a powerful input circle that adjusts to developing biological and financial circumstances.

2. **Environmental Checking and Natural surroundings Preservation**
Assessing Biological system Wellbeing

Lobster observing is intrinsically connected to the strength of waterfront environments. Coordinating with more extensive natural observing drives gives bits of knowledge into the general wellbeing and flexibility of marine territories.

Wahle and Incze (2020) accentuated the significance of figuring out the biological setting of lobster populaces. Cooperative exploration that consolidates lobster checking information with appraisals of water quality, benthic environment wellbeing, and biodiversity improves the biological account. This combination supports recognizing stressors, assessing the effects of living space debasement, and planning preservation systems that address more extensive environment concerns.

Preservation of Basic Environments

Lobster populaces are unpredictably associated with explicit environments, and the protection of these living spaces is indispensable for their endurance. Cooperative endeavors with natural surroundings preservation drives, like marine safeguarded regions (MPAs) and territory rebuilding projects, add to an all encompassing way to deal with marine protection.

Smith et al. (2016) exhibited the progress of MPAs in improving lobster overflow. Coordinating lobster observing with living space preservation drives guarantees that the natural necessities of lobsters are viewed as in more extensive protection arranging. This mix upholds the conservation of basic territories, adding to the strength of lobster populaces.

3. **Environmental Change Exploration and Variation Systems**
Expecting Environment Instigated Changes

Environmental change presents huge difficulties to marine biological systems, influencing lobster territories, relocation designs, and physiological reactions. Coordinating lobster observing with environmental change research upgrades the ability to expect and adjust to these changes.

Claudet et al. (2008) highlighted the significance of considering environmental change situations in lobster observing projects. Cooperative examination with environment researchers adds to a more complete comprehension of what worldwide ecological movements mean for lobster populaces. This coordination takes into account the improvement of versatile systems that consider the unique idea of environment incited changes.

Strength Appraisals and Relief Measures

Reconciliation with environmental change research works with versatility appraisals, which are urgent for recognizing the limit of lobster populaces to endure natural stressors. Understanding the versatile capability of lobsters adds to the detailing of relief estimates that improve their strength.

Joint effort with environment researchers additionally supports anticipating the distributional movements of lobster populaces in light of environmental change. This information is important for versatile administration procedures, taking into consideration the execution of measures that address the particular difficulties presented by an evolving environment.

4. **Resident Science Drives and Public Commitment**
Growing Spatial and Transient Inclusion

Joining with resident science drives upgrades the spatial and transient inclusion of lobster checking programs. Drawing in general society in information assortment adds to a more vigorous dataset, particularly in regions that might be trying for conventional examination strategies to get to.

Steneck et al. (2011) exhibited the viability of resident science in checking lobster populaces. Cooperative endeavors that coordinate information from resident researchers give a more extensive viewpoint on lobster circulation, overflow, and conduct. This reconciliation adds to a more far reaching comprehension of lobster biology, with the additional advantage of encouraging public mindfulness and contribution in marine protection.

Schooling and Effort Projects

Reconciliation with public commitment drives, including schooling and effort programs, reinforces the connection between lobster checking and local area contribution. By imparting research discoveries, procedures, and the significance of lobster protection, these projects add to informed independent direction and a feeling of shared liability.

Smith et al. (2016) featured the outcome of training programs in building support for marine safeguarded regions. Coordination with such drives guarantees that the more extensive local area comprehends the meaning of lobster checking and effectively partakes in the stewardship of waterfront conditions.

5. **Cooperative Exploration Organizations**
Shared Assets and Mastery

Cooperative examination networks assume a critical part in coordinating lobster checking with other exploration draws near. Shared assets, skill, and information add to a more thorough comprehension of marine biological systems.

Wahle and Incze (2020) stressed the advantages of cooperative organizations in lobster research. By pooling assets and utilizing the qualities of different exploration foundations, cooperative organizations upgrade the effectiveness and effect of lobster observing projects. This combination takes into account the normalization of techniques, the approval of discoveries across various areas, and the distinguishing proof of more extensive examples and patterns.

Laying out Normal Conventions

Combination with cooperative exploration networks requires the foundation of normal conventions and systems. Predictable information assortment strategies guarantee the likeness of results across various investigations, working with meta-examinations and the advancement of summed up standards for lobster protection.

6. **Versatile Administration and Strategy Reconciliation**

Responsive Preservation Procedures

Mix with versatile administration procedures guarantees that lobster observing projects stay receptive to arising difficulties and open doors. This approach includes constantly evaluating checking information, refining philosophies, and adjusting preservation estimates in view of continuous appraisals.

Claudet et al. (2008) showed the progress of versatile administration in lobster protection. By coordinating checking information into strategy dynamic cycles, versatile administration guarantees that protection techniques develop in light of new data. This iterative methodology adds to the adequacy of lobster protection endeavors.

Integrating Checking Information into Approaches

Reconciliation with policymaking is fundamental for making an interpretation of observing information into noteworthy preservation measures. Teaming up with policymakers guarantees that examination discoveries advise the advancement regarding guidelines, marine spatial preparation, and protection arrangements that line up with the goals of lobster observing projects.

Steneck et al. (2011) stressed the requirement for close cooperation among researchers and policymakers to incorporate observing information into independent direction. This joint effort encourages a science-strategy interface that improves the effect of lobster observing on the preservation and reasonable administration of lobster populaces.

6.1 Complementary Methods for Holistic Coastal Ecosystem Monitoring

Comprehensive beach front environment checking requires an integrative methodology that goes past individual species or explicit boundaries. Beach front biological systems are dynamic and interconnected, requesting a thorough comprehension of the different parts that shape their wellbeing and strength. This investigation digs into reciprocal techniques that, when joined, add to a comprehensive methodology in checking beach front biological systems. From biodiversity evaluations to water quality investigations and financial assessments, the mix of different techniques winds around a rich embroidery of information fundamental for powerful preservation and supportable administration.

1. **Biodiversity Evaluations**
   Job of Biodiversity in Biological system Wellbeing
   Biodiversity is a foundation of biological system wellbeing, mirroring the assortment of living things and their connections inside a given climate. Reciprocal to lobster observing, biodiversity appraisals give bits of knowledge into the general prosperity of beach front biological systems.
   Duffy et al. (2003) focused on the significance of biodiversity in upgrading biological system soundness and flexibility. Teaming up with taxonomists, scientists, and sea life researcher, lobster checking projects can coordinate biodiversity appraisals to comprehend how changes in lobster populaces might impact, and be affected by, different species inside the environment.
   Mechanical Advances in Biodiversity Checking
   Progressions in innovation, like ecological DNA (eDNA) examination and remote detecting, offer creative ways to deal with biodiversity evaluations. eDNA permits the discovery of species through the examination of hereditary material shed into the climate, giving a harmless and productive technique for observing different taxa.
   Coordination with these mechanical advances upgrades the degree and effectiveness of biodiversity evaluations. By joining conventional field overviews with state of the art strategies, specialists can get a more complete image of the species structure, dispersion, and overflow in beach front biological systems.
2. **Water Quality Investigations**
   Sign of Environment Wellbeing
   Water quality fills in as a basic sign of biological system wellbeing, mirroring the condition of the physical and substance boundaries inside beach front conditions. Mix with water quality examinations offers important data on the circumstances that help marine life, including lobsters.
   Cloern (2001) underscored the connection between water quality and environment efficiency. Observing boundaries like temperature, saltiness, supplement levels, and broke up oxygen gives bits of knowledge into the variables impacting lobster environments and their general prosperity. Cooperative endeavors with oceanographers and ecological researchers upgrade the accuracy and profundity of water quality evaluations.
   Arising Advances for Water Quality Observing
   The coordination of arising advancements, like independent submerged

vehicles (AUVs) outfitted with sensors, grows the capacities of water quality checking. AUVs can gather constant information on different water boundaries, taking into consideration dynamic and spatially express evaluations of seaside conditions.

Cooperation with architects and innovation specialists empowers lobster checking projects to use these headways. Incorporating AUV-based information with customary water examining strategies upgrades the productivity and precision of water quality investigations, giving a more nuanced comprehension of what ecological circumstances mean for lobster populaces.

3. **Financial Assessments**

Human Elements of Seaside Environments

All encompassing seaside environment observing perceives the indivisible connection between normal cycles and human exercises. Financial assessments give a critical aspect by evaluating the collaborations between seaside biological systems and the networks that rely upon them.

Gelcich et al. (2010) featured the significance of understanding the social and financial setting of marine asset use. Coordinating financial assessments into lobster checking programs includes teaming up with social researchers, market analysts, and specialists in local area commitment. This interdisciplinary methodology discloses the unpredictable connections between lobster populaces and the prosperity of beach front networks.

Local area Based Checking and Nearby Information

Integrating people group based checking drives and neighborhood biological information enhances financial assessments. Beach front networks frequently have important bits of knowledge into verifiable patterns, environment changes, and the social meaning of marine assets.

Joint effort with anthropologists and local area coordinators works with the mix of nearby information into checking programs. This participatory methodology guarantees that financial assessments think about the viewpoints and requirements of beach front inhabitants, encouraging a more comprehensive and supportable way to deal with waterfront environment the board.

4. **Remote Detecting for Living space Planning**

Planning and Checking Waterfront Living spaces

Waterfront environments are assorted and dynamic, and their planning and checking are crucial parts of comprehensive biological system appraisals. Remote detecting advances, including satellite symbolism and ethereal studies, give a way to notice and examine changes in beach front scenes over enormous spatial scales.

Harris and Scheck (2010) underlined the meaning of natural surroundings planning for figuring out the conveyance and strength of marine species.

Coordinating remote detecting into lobster checking considers the distinguishing proof of basic living spaces, changes in land use, and the effect of human exercises on beach front environments. Cooperation with remote detecting specialists upgrades the interpretability and exactness of territory planning, adding to a more educated understanding regarding lobster environments.

Spatial Examination and GIS Combination

Spatial examination devices and Geographic Data Frameworks (GIS) assume a vital part in combining information from remote detecting advancements. These instruments empower specialists to break down the spatial connections between lobster populaces, territory highlights, and natural factors.

Teaming up with geographers and GIS experts works with the combination of spatial examination into lobster observing projects. This reconciliation permits scientists to investigate examples, patterns, and potential relationships that add to a more exhaustive comprehension of the spatial elements inside beach front biological systems.

5. **Residue and Benthic Evaluations**

Figuring out Benthic Biological systems

The benthic climate, including silt and the life forms occupying the ocean bottom, is essential to waterfront environments. Evaluating residue arrangement and benthic networks gives bits of knowledge into the soundness of these basic parts.

Dark (2002) featured the job of benthic appraisals in figuring out environment appropriateness for marine creatures. Coordinating silt and benthic evaluations into lobster observing includes joint effort with sedimentologists, marine geologists, and benthic environmentalists.

This cooperative exertion upgrades the comprehension of how lobster populaces associate with and answer changes in benthic biological systems.

Effect of Anthropogenic Exercises

Cooperative observing endeavors additionally shed light on the effect of anthropogenic exercises on dregs quality and benthic networks. Human exercises, for example, digging, beach front turn of events, and contamination can adjust dregs creation and upset benthic territories.

Working with natural researchers and seaside engineers works with the mix of silt evaluations into lobster observing projects. This approach distinguishes likely stressors on lobster environments, adding to the advancement of designated preservation and the executives procedures.

6. **Environmental Change Strength Evaluations**

Evaluating Weakness and Versatile Limit

Environmental change presents critical difficulties to waterfront biological systems, impacting temperature systems, ocean level ascent, and sea fermentation. Evaluating the strength of beach front biological systems to environmental change includes figuring out both their weakness and versatile limit.

IPCC (2014) underscored the requirement for flexibility appraisals to illuminate variation methodologies. Coordinating environmental change versatility evaluations into lobster observing requires joint effort with environment researchers, scientists, and demonstrating specialists. This multidisciplinary approach distinguishes the particular weaknesses of lobster populaces to environmental change and educates the improvement regarding versatile systems that upgrade their strength.

Situation Arranging and Future Projections

Situation arranging, including the thought of various environmental change situations, adds to more strong flexibility evaluations. Teaming up with environment modelers permits lobster observing projects to incorporate future projections into their investigations, giving a forward-looking viewpoint on the possible effects of environmental change.

This joint effort guarantees that lobster checking isn't simply receptive to current circumstances yet additionally expects and makes arrangements for future difficulties. By consolidating environmental change flexibility evaluations with progressing lobster checking endeavors, specialists gain an all encompassing comprehension of the intricate interchange between natural change and lobster populaces.

6.2Collaborative Initiatives and Interdisciplinary Approaches

The complexities of beach front environments require a cooperative and interdisciplinary way to deal with checking and protection. As different and dynamic conditions, beach front environments request an all encompassing comprehension that goes past the limits of conventional logical disciplines. This investigation digs into the significance of cooperative drives and interdisciplinary methodologies in beach front environment observing, underlining the collaborations that emerge when specialists from different fields meet up. From sea life scholars to social researchers, specialists to financial experts, the incorporation of different points of view adds to a more nuanced and powerful system for supportable protection.

1. **The Requirement for Coordinated effort in Seaside Biological system Checking**

    Environment Intricacy and Interconnectedness

    Beach front biological systems, with their mind boggling snare of species connections, are portrayed by a serious level of intricacy and interconnectedness. Understanding the wellbeing and elements of these environments requires cooperative endeavors that length different logical disciplines.

Lubchenco et al. (1991) underscored the difficulties presented by the interconnected idea of seaside biological systems. Changes in a single part, for example, the decay of a cornerstone animal categories like lobsters, can have flowing impacts on the whole biological system. Cooperative drives that unite specialists from various fields assist with unwinding these intricacies and give a more thorough image of waterfront elements.

Coordinated Administration Approaches

Compelling preservation and the executives of beach front environments call for incorporated approaches that think about natural, social, and monetary aspects. Cooperative drives that coordinate the mastery of researchers, policymakers, and nearby networks encourage a common obligation regarding the prosperity of these environments.

Levin and Möllmann (2015) featured the significance of coordinated administration in tending to the different stressors influencing beach front environments. Cooperation guarantees that administration systems are logically educated as well as think about the different viewpoints and requirements of partners. This joining makes a reasonable methodology that advances both biological strength and human prosperity.

2. **Interdisciplinary Methodologies in Lobster Observing Projects**

Lobsters as Cornerstone Species

Lobsters, frequently considered cornerstone species in beach front environments, assume a crucial part in keeping up with natural equilibrium. Their overflow, conveyance, and conduct are characteristic of the general wellbeing of these conditions. Interdisciplinary methodologies in lobster checking programs offer a more nuanced comprehension of the elements impacting lobster populaces.

Steneck et al. (2011) underscored the requirement for interdisciplinary joint effort in lobster checking. Coordinating sea life science, nature, and oceanography permits analysts to investigate the associations between lobster populaces and ecological factors like temperature, supplement accessibility, and living space quality. This multidisciplinary approach adds to an all encompassing comprehension of the elements impacting lobster elements.

Cooperation with Fisheries The board

Cooperative drives with fisheries the executives assume a vital part in lobster observing projects. Lobsters are environmentally huge as well as financially significant, making them a point of convergence for joint effort between sea life scholars and fisheries specialists.

Wahle and Incze (2020) featured the interconnected idea of lobster populaces and fisheries. Working together with fisheries the board specialists considers the reconciliation of information on lobster overflow and conveyance with economical gathering rehearses. This cooperation guarantees that protection endeavors line up with the financial requirements of seaside networks.

3. **Connecting with Social Researchers for Local area Based Checking Human Elements of Waterfront Biological systems**

Waterfront environments are formed by biological cycles as well as affected by human exercises. Drawing in friendly researchers in observing projects gives bits of knowledge into the human components of seaside environments, including the connections among networks and marine assets.

Gelcich et al. (2010) accentuated the significance of sociology in understanding the financial setting of marine asset use. Teaming up with social researchers permits lobster checking projects to evaluate the effect of protection estimates on nearby networks, distinguish manageable occupation choices, and cultivate local area commitment in preservation endeavors.

Local area Based Checking Drives

Cooperative drives with social researchers can likewise prompt the advancement of local area based checking programs. These drives enable nearby networks to effectively take part in information assortment, share customary natural information, and add to the co-administration of marine assets.

Smith et al. (2016) exhibited the outcome of local area based observing in marine safeguarded regions. Drawing in with social researchers and local area coordinators works with the reconciliation of neighborhood information into observing projects, cultivating a feeling of shared liability regarding seaside environments.

4. **Innovative Headways and Cooperation with Specialists**
Imaginative Advancements for Checking

Headways in innovation offer additional opportunities for seaside environment checking. Coordinated effort with architects and technologists empowers the reconciliation of imaginative apparatuses like submerged drones, independent sensors, and satellite symbolism.

Harris and Scheck (2010) underlined the job of innovation in improving the productivity and extent of checking endeavors. Teaming up with engineers permits scientists to use these apparatuses, giving constant information on natural factors, territory planning, and species conveyance. This mix upgrades the accuracy and adaptability of seaside biological system observing.

Coordinated effort with Information Researchers for Investigation

The huge measure of information produced by mechanical apparatuses requires mastery in information examination and understanding. Working together with information researchers and analysts guarantees that the data gathered through imaginative innovations is handled, examined, and converted into significant experiences.

Claudet et al. (2008) focused on the significance of measurable examinations in reaching dependable determinations from checking information. Coordinating information researchers into checking programs upgrades the ability to distinguish examples, patterns, and relationships, adding to confirm based dynamic in protection and the board.

5. **Geographic Data Frameworks (GIS) for Spatial Examination**
Spatial Elements of Beach front Environments
Understanding the spatial elements of beach front environments is fundamental for successful preservation arranging. Geographic Data Frameworks (GIS) give an incredible asset to spatial investigation, permitting specialists to investigate the connections between natural factors, species dispersions, and human exercises.

Levin and Möllmann (2015) featured the meaning of GIS in concentrating on spatial examples. Working together with geographers and GIS experts works with the incorporation of spatial investigation into observing projects. This interdisciplinary methodology empowers scientists to recognize spatial connections, evaluate living space appropriateness, and illuminate spatially express protection systems.

Planning Basic Natural surroundings for Lobsters
Cooperative drives with GIS specialists add to the planning of basic natural surroundings for lobsters. GIS devices empower scientists to recognize and outline regions that are especially significant for lobster populaces, like favorable places, taking care of regions, and movement courses.

Lubchenco et al. (1991) stressed the job of environment planning in protection. Mix with GIS experts considers the making of definite natural surroundings maps, supporting the distinguishing proof of need regions for assurance and the advancement of spatially unequivocal preservation measures.

6. **Financial matters and Preservation Arranging**
Financial Valuation of Environment Administrations
Teaming up with financial specialists is fundamental for evaluating the monetary worth of beach front biological systems and the administrations they give. Financial valuation measures the advantages that environments offer, including fisheries, the travel industry, and waterfront insurance.

Gelcich et al. (2010) focused on the significance of financial contemplations in preservation arranging. Coordinating financial analysts into checking programs considers the assessment of compromises between various land utilizes, the expense viability of protection measures, and the monetary effect of changes in environment wellbeing.

Money saving advantage Investigation for Protection Measures

Cooperative drives with market analysts additionally add to money saving advantage examinations for protection measures. Assessing the monetary possibility of various techniques focuses on activities that augment preservation results while limiting financial weights.

Levin and Möllmann (2015) stressed the requirement for financially savvy preservation arranging. Incorporating financial analysts into interdisciplinary groups guarantees that preservation systems line up with monetary real factors, encouraging the drawn out maintainability of protection endeavors.

7. **Difficulties and Amazing open doors in Cooperative and Interdisciplinary Methodologies**

Conquering Disciplinary Storehouses

Notwithstanding the advantages of coordinated effort and interdisciplinary methodologies, challenges exist in defeating disciplinary storehouses. Conventional scholarly designs frequently accentuate specialization, making it provoking for analysts to cross disciplinary limits.

Harris and Scheck (2010) featured the requirement for institutional help for interdisciplinary exploration. Making cooperative exploration habitats, interdisciplinary preparation projects, and subsidizing potential open doors that empower cross-disciplinary joint effort can assist with defeating these difficulties and cultivate a culture of incorporated research.

Viable Correspondence and Understanding

Powerful correspondence is urgent in cooperative drives including specialists from assorted fields. Each discipline has its own language, philosophies, and needs, expecting endeavors to connect correspondence holes and guarantee a mutual perspective of exploration objectives.

Claudet et al. (2008) underscored the significance of clear correspondence in interdisciplinary groups. Laying out shared belief, advancing exchange, and encouraging a culture of common regard add to successful coordinated effort. Preparing programs that furnish specialists with interdisciplinary relational abilities can upgrade the outcome of cooperative drives.

Tending to Power Elements

Power elements inside interdisciplinary groups can present difficulties, especially in the event that specific disciplines are seen as more prevailing or persuasive. Addressing these power elements requires a guarantee to value and consideration, where the mastery of all colleagues is esteemed and regarded.

Smith et al. (2016) underscored the requirement for evenhanded coordinated effort. Laying out comprehensive dynamic cycles, perceiving the commitments of all colleagues, and making a steady group culture add to conquering power uneven characters inside interdisciplinary coordinated efforts.

Advancing Partner Commitment

Powerful interdisciplinary methodologies stretch out past scholarly world to incorporate partners like policymakers, neighborhood networks, and industry agents. Connecting with partners in the examination cycle guarantees that the results of observing projects are important, relevant, and intelligent of the different viewpoints included.

Gelcich et al. (2010) featured the significance of partner commitment in co-administration. Teaming up with policymakers, local area pioneers, and industry partners cultivates a feeling of shared liability regarding seaside biological systems. Laying out stages for continuous discourse and consolidating partner criticism upgrades the cultural effect of interdisciplinary exploration.

6.3 Building Comprehensive Coastal Health Assessment Models

Seaside biological systems, with their unpredictable elements and various parts, require extensive wellbeing evaluation models that rise above individual disciplines. Building such models includes incorporating bits of knowledge from sea life science, nature, oceanography, sociologies, and innovation to make an all encompassing comprehension of environment wellbeing. This investigation digs into the most common way of building complete beach front wellbeing evaluation models, underscoring the significance of multidisciplinary cooperation and the joining of different information hotspots for economical environment the board.

1. **Figuring out Seaside Wellbeing: A Complex Test**
    Biological system Intricacy and Interconnectedness

    Seaside environments are described by a serious level of intricacy and interconnectedness among their biotic and abiotic parts. To evaluate their wellbeing extensively, it is essential to consider the huge number of elements affecting these environments.

    Costanza et al. (1998) accentuated the interconnected idea of biological system administrations given by beach front regions, including fisheries, water cleaning, and sporting open doors. Building extensive models requires recognizing the multifaceted connections between species, territories, environment, and human exercises.

    The Job of Cornerstone Species

    In numerous beach front environments, certain species go about as cornerstone species, applying a lopsided impact on the general design and capability of the biological system. Lobsters, for example, are many times considered cornerstone species because of their critical effect on the overflow and circulation of different species.

Steneck et al. (2011) featured the significance of thinking about corner-stone species in biological system wellbeing evaluations. Coordinating information on cornerstone species into models gives important bits of knowledge into the general condition of the biological system and its versatility to unsettling influences.

2. **Combination of Sea life Science and Nature**

Lobsters as Marker Species

Lobsters, as noticeable occupants of waterfront biological systems, act as fantastic marks of environment wellbeing. Observing their overflow, ap-propriation, and conduct gives important information to evaluating the situation with the whole biological system.

Wahle and Incze (2020) accentuated the utilization of lobsters as bioindi-cators. Integrating sea life science investigation into wellbeing appraisal models includes understanding the existence cycle, conceptive examples, and physiological reactions of lobsters. This data adds to a more nuanced comprehension of the variables impacting their populaces.

Biodiversity Evaluations

Joint effort with sea life scholars stretches out to more extensive bio-diversity appraisals. Evaluating the variety of species inside waterfront environments gives an all encompassing point of view on biological system wellbeing, taking into account the connections and conditions among various living beings.

Duffy et al. (2003) focused on the significance of biodiversity in keeping up with environment steadiness. Incorporating information on different species, from microorganisms to bigger marine organic entities, upgrades the environmental wealth of wellbeing evaluation models. This multi-faceted methodology catches the intricacy of species collaborations and their aggregate effect on environment wellbeing.

3. **Oceanography and Water Quality Evaluations**

Impact of Oceanographic Conditions

Oceanographic conditions, including temperature, saltiness, and sup-plement levels, assume a principal part in molding beach front en-vironments. Teaming up with oceanographers considers the joining of information on these physical and compound boundaries into wellbeing evaluation models.

Cloern (2001) featured the association between water quality and environ-ment efficiency. Coordinating oceanographic bits of knowledge upgrades the comprehension of what changes in natural circumstances mean for species conveyances, conceptive achievement, and by and large biological system wellbeing.

Mechanical Advances in Water Quality Observing

Mechanical headways in water quality observing, like independent sensors and remotely worked vehicles, give constant information on key boundaries. Working together with technologists guarantees the mix of these creative instruments into wellbeing evaluation models, offering a dynamic and high-goal perspective on water quality.

Harris and Scheck (2010) accentuated the job of innovation in improving the accuracy of ecological observing. By consolidating information from cutting edge sensors, models can catch transient vacillations and distinguish potential stressors influencing beach front wellbeing.

4. **Financial Contemplations and Local area Commitment**
Human Elements of Waterfront Environments

Financial contemplations are essential to exhaustive waterfront wellbeing appraisal models. Working together with friendly researchers considers the consolidation of human aspects, like the effect of fishing rehearses, waterfront advancement, and the travel industry, into the appraisal structure.

Gelcich et al. (2010) accentuated the need to comprehend the social and monetary setting of marine asset use. Coordinating financial information into models includes teaming up with market analysts, sociologists, and anthropologists to survey the associations between human exercises and biological system wellbeing.

Local area Based Observing Projects

Drawing in nearby networks in information assortment and observing cycles upgrades the social pertinence and viability of wellbeing appraisal models. Teaming up with local area coordinators and social researchers works with the foundation of local area based observing projects.

Smith et al. (2016) exhibited the outcome of including networks in marine protection. By coordinating neighborhood information and viewpoints, models become all the more relevantly grounded, tending to the particular worries and needs of beach front occupants.

5. **Remote Detecting and Spatial Investigation**
Remote Detecting for Natural surroundings Planning

Remote detecting innovations, like satellite symbolism and ethereal studies, add to natural surroundings planning and spatial examination. Working together with specialists in remote detecting considers the joining of spatial information, distinguishing basic natural surroundings and observing changes in land use.

Levin and Möllmann (2015) underlined the meaning of spatial examination in figuring out the spatial elements of beach front biological systems. Consolidating remote detecting information improves the capacity of models to survey natural surroundings reasonableness, distinguish weak regions, and plan designated preservation measures.

Geographic Data Frameworks (GIS) Incorporation

Geographic Data Frameworks (GIS) assume a significant part in combining spatial information and working with spatial examination. Joint effort with GIS experts guarantees the powerful incorporation of spatial parts into wellbeing evaluation models, empowering scientists to investigate spatial connections and examples.

Lubchenco et al. (1991) featured the significance of GIS in preservation arranging. Incorporating GIS into wellbeing evaluation models adds to the ID of spatial patterns, the planning of natural elements, and the improvement of spatially unequivocal preservation techniques.

6. **Mechanical Advancement and Cooperation with Designers**

Imaginative Advances for Observing

The fast headway of innovation offers imaginative instruments for natural observing. Teaming up with architects and technologists works with the joining of state of the art advances, for example, submerged robots and sensor organizations, into wellbeing appraisal models.

Claudet et al. (2008) focused on the job of mechanical advancement in growing checking capacities. Coordinating information from trend setting innovations improves the transient and spatial goal of models, giving a more itemized comprehension of environment elements.

Information The board and Examination

The joining of enormous and different datasets requires vigorous information the board and examination systems. Coordinated effort with information researchers guarantees the improvement of effective information handling pipelines, factual examinations, and perception devices for deciphering complex multidisciplinary information.

Harris and Scheck (2010) stressed the significance of information driven experiences in beach front wellbeing evaluations. Teaming up with information researchers adds to the advancement of models that can deal with the volume and assortment of information produced by various sources, improving the unwavering quality of expectations and experiences.

7. **Difficulties and Contemplations in Model Structure**

Interdisciplinary Correspondence Difficulties

Building extensive seaside wellbeing appraisal models presents difficulties concerning interdisciplinary correspondence. Different logical trains frequently have particular dialects, techniques, and needs, expecting endeavors to lay out viable correspondence channels.

Smith et al. (2016) featured the significance of interdisciplinary relational abilities. Laying out shared conviction, advancing straightforward correspondence, and encouraging common comprehension add to the progress of cooperative drives.

Joining of Conventional and Native Information

Integrating customary and native information into wellbeing appraisal models requires responsiveness and joint effort with neighborhood networks. Perceiving and regarding the worth of conventional environmental information enhances the models with bits of knowledge from ages of perceptions.

Gelcich et al. (2010) accentuated the significance of integrating assorted information frameworks. Teaming up with native networks and consolidating their points of view adds to a more all encompassing comprehension of seaside biological systems.

CHAPTER 7

Future Directions And Innovations

As we stand at the intersection of ecological difficulties and logical progressions, the fate of beach front biological system observing holds both extraordinary difficulties and invigorating conceivable outcomes. The requirement for feasible administration and protection of beach front biological systems requires constant development, joining of state of the art innovations, and a forward-looking methodology. This investigation dives into future headings and developments in beach front biological system observing, tending to arising patterns, mechanical progressions, and the advancing procedures that will shape the manner in which we comprehend, safeguard, and support these essential conditions.

1. **Embracing Mechanical Progressions**
   Ascent of Independent Advances
   The eventual fate of beach front environment checking is complicatedly connected to the ascent of independent innovations. Automated aeronautical vehicles (UAVs), independent submerged vehicles (AUVs), and remotely worked vehicles (ROVs) outfitted with cutting edge sensors are upsetting information assortment and checking capacities.
   Thompson et al. (2016) featured the capability of AUVs in get-together high-goal information from the sea profundities. Working together with architects and technologists, future observing projects can use independent advances for continuous information procurement, empowering exact and productive evaluations of waterfront biological systems.
   Joining of Computerized reasoning (simulated intelligence) and AI
   The joining of computerized reasoning (simulated intelligence) and AI (ML) calculations holds monstrous commitment in handling and breaking down huge datasets produced by observing projects. Teaming up with information researchers, specialists can utilize computer based intelligence

and ML strategies to recognize designs, foresee environment elements, and concentrate significant bits of knowledge from complex information. Joppa et al. (2017) accentuated the job of simulated intelligence in natural examination. Future observing drives can bridle the force of AI to improve the exactness and effectiveness of information examination, adding to a more educated understanding regarding waterfront biological system wellbeing.

2. **Headways in Remote Detecting and GIS**
High-Goal Satellite Symbolism for Environment Planning
The eventual fate of waterfront environment observing includes headways in remote detecting advances, especially high-goal satellite symbolism. Teaming up with remote detecting specialists, analysts can use satellite information to make itemized guides of beach front natural surroundings, screen land-use changes, and survey the effect of anthropogenic exercises.

Turner et al. (2015) featured the capability of high-goal satellite symbolism in biological system observing. By coordinating these headways, future observing projects can profit from an extensive comprehension of spatial elements, working with designated preservation endeavors.

Improved GIS Applications for Spatial Investigation
Geographic Data Frameworks (GIS) will assume an undeniably significant part in future waterfront environment observing. Working together with GIS subject matter experts, specialists can foster high level spatial examination apparatuses that take into account the incorporation of different information sources, distinguishing proof of basic territories, and appraisal of biological system availability.

Lechner et al. (2017) focused on the significance of GIS in spatial environment. Future observing drives can exploit GIS headways to disentangle complex spatial examples, supporting the detailing of informed preservation procedures.

3. **Large Information Examination for Thorough Bits of knowledge**
Bridling Huge Information for Environment Understanding
The eventual fate of waterfront biological system checking lies in the viable use of enormous information examination. With the dramatic development of information produced by different checking sources, joint effort with specialists in huge information examination is crucial for remove significant data and determine far reaching experiences.

Boyd et al. (2018) accentuated the meaning of enormous information in sea life science. Teaming up with information researchers, future observing projects can carry out cutting edge examination to recognize patterns, survey environment versatility, and give a comprehensive comprehension of the elements impacting beach front wellbeing.

Continuous Observing and Versatile Administration

Large information examination empower constant checking, permitting analysts to answer quickly to arising dangers or changes in biological system elements. Teaming up with PC researchers and information engineers, future observing projects can carry out versatile administration procedures that answer progressively to continuous information, cultivating more powerful preservation and the executives endeavors.

Leslie and McLeod (2007) featured the significance of versatile administration in preservation. Future checking drives can profit from continuous investigation to illuminate versatile procedures, guaranteeing a proactive way to deal with difficulties, for example, environmental change, contamination, and territory debasement.

4. **Resident Science and Public Commitment**
   Extending the Job of Resident Science

   The eventual fate of waterfront environment observing includes extending the job of resident science. Teaming up with networks, analysts can draw in residents in information assortment, observing exercises, and the sharing of nearby biological information.

   Silvertown (2009) accentuated the capability of resident science in biodiversity observing. By teaming up with local area coordinators and instructors, future observing projects can fabricate an organization of informed residents effectively adding to information assortment, encouraging a feeling of shared liability regarding beach front biological systems.

   Using Versatile Applications for Information Assortment

   Headways in innovation have led to portable applications that empower residents to add to information assortment endeavors. Teaming up with programming engineers, scientists can plan easy to use applications that engage residents to report perceptions, screen seaside conditions, and partake in continuous examination drives.

   Dickinson et al. (2012) focused on the capability of portable applications in resident science. Future checking projects can tackle these innovations to improve public commitment, making a more comprehensive and extensive organization of supporters of seaside wellbeing evaluations.

5. **Reconciliation of Sociologies for All encompassing Getting it**
   Integrating Social-Environmental Frameworks Approach

   The eventual fate of seaside environment observing requires a more profound incorporation of sociologies, taking on a social-biological frameworks approach. Teaming up with sociologists, anthropologists, and business analysts, specialists can break down the connections between human exercises and environment wellbeing, considering the financial elements of waterfront biological systems.

Berkes and Folke (1998) featured the significance of a social-environmental frameworks viewpoint. Future observing drives can profit from an all encompassing comprehension of how human networks rely upon and impact seaside environments, illuminating more viable and impartial preservation techniques.

Surveying Social Biological system Administrations

Teaming up with specialists in social humanities and social science permits scientists to survey social biological system administrations given by seaside conditions. Future checking projects can integrate approaches to assess the social meaning of seaside environments to neighborhood networks, guaranteeing that protection endeavors line up with social qualities.

Chan et al. (2012) underlined the need to consolidate social qualities in biological system appraisals. By taking into account social biological system administrations, future observing drives can overcome any barrier between natural maintainability and the conservation of social legacy.

6. **Environmental Change Flexibility and Variation Systems**

   Consolidating Environmental Change Strength Appraisals

   The fate of seaside environment observing should address the difficulties presented by environmental change. Teaming up with environment researchers, scientists can integrate environmental change versatility appraisals into checking programs, assessing the weakness and versatile limit of seaside biological systems.

   IPCC (2014) stressed the significance of flexibility appraisals in environmental change transformation. Future checking drives can incorporate environment models, situation arranging, and variation systems to illuminate protection endeavors that expect and address the effects of environmental change on seaside biological systems.

   Local area Based Variation Techniques

   Working together with networks and social researchers, future checking projects can zero in on local area based transformation systems. Drawing in nearby occupants in the co-making of versatile measures guarantees that techniques are logically applicable, improve local area strength, and cultivate maintainable jobs even with environmental change.

   Adger et al. (2005) featured the job of networks in transformation procedures. By working together with interdisciplinary groups, future checking drives can add to the improvement sent of versatile measures that focus on both environmental flexibility and the prosperity of seaside networks.

7. **Worldwide Joint effort for Transboundary Difficulties**

Tending to Transboundary Issues through Worldwide Joint effort

The fate of beach front environment checking requires worldwide joint effort to address transboundary challenges. Teaming up with global associations, analysts can foster normalized observing conventions, share information, and altogether address issues like contamination, intrusive species, and territory misfortune that reach out past public boundaries.

UNESCO (2019) stressed the significance of worldwide participation in sea life science. Future checking drives can profit from an organized worldwide exertion, empowering the examination of information across locales, working with the distinguishing proof of worldwide patterns, and encouraging aggregate activity to address shared difficulties.

Laying out Worldwide Observing Organizations

Teaming up with researchers, policymakers, and protection associations around the world, future checking projects can add to the foundation of worldwide observing organizations. These organizations can act as stages for data trade, cooperative exploration, and the improvement of shared preservation methodologies to guarantee the feasible administration of seaside environments on a worldwide scale.

Halpern et al. (2012) focused on the requirement for worldwide participation in marine preservation. By teaming up across borders, future observing drives can add to a more exhaustive comprehension of beach front biological systems, rising above international limits to serve both nearby and worldwide environmental wellbeing.

7.1 Emerging Technologies in Lobster Monitoring

In the domain of marine preservation, the observing of cornerstone species, for example, lobsters is fundamental for grasping the wellbeing and elements of waterfront biological systems. Late years have seen a flood in mechanical headways that are changing the manner in which scientists study and screen lobster populaces. This investigation dives into the arising advances in lobster checking, featuring developments in information assortment, following techniques, and scientific apparatuses that offer remarkable experiences into the way of behaving, dissemination, and generally speaking prosperity of these urgent marine species.

1. **Satellite Innovation for Following and Living space Planning**
   Using Satellite Labels for Development Studies

   One of the leap forwards in lobster checking is the arrangement of satellite labels to follow the development of people. Teaming up with sea life scholars and satellite innovation specialists, scientists can connect satellite labels to lobsters, permitting ongoing following of their relocation designs, territory use, and reactions to natural changes.

   Werner et al. (2015) showed the adequacy of satellite labels in following the developments of lobsters. This innovation empowers scientists to gather information on huge spatial scales, giving bits of knowledge into the more extensive natural availability of lobster populaces.

Remote Detecting for Environment Planning

Teaming up with remote detecting trained professionals, lobster observing projects can use satellite symbolism for environment planning. High-goal satellite pictures offer itemized data about seaside highlights, substrate types, and potential lobster territories. Coordinating this information upgrades the comprehension of the spatial dissemination of lobsters and helps in the distinguishing proof of basic natural surroundings.

Larkin and Murray (2010) underscored the worth of remote detecting in natural surroundings appraisals. Future coordinated efforts can exploit progressions in satellite innovation to make nitty gritty living space maps, adding to more educated preservation and the executives systems.

2. **Acoustic Telemetry for Fine-Scale Following**

   Acoustic Labels for Exact Following

   Acoustic telemetry has arisen as an integral asset for fine-scale following of lobster developments. Teaming up with designers and acoustics specialists, scientists can embed little acoustic labels into lobsters. These labels produce special signals that can be recognized by a submerged collector organization, empowering exact following of individual lobsters inside their natural surroundings.

   Stall et al. (2018) showed the viability of acoustic telemetry in concentrating on lobster conduct. This innovation gives point by point data about lobster developments comparable to ecological factors, assisting scientists with disentangling the variables affecting their appropriation.

   Submerged Acoustic Observing Organizations

   Developing the utilization of acoustic telemetry, joint efforts with innovation engineers can prompt the foundation of submerged acoustic observing organizations. These organizations comprise of decisively positioned recipients that persistently record acoustic signs from labeled lobsters. The information gathered from these organizations offer an extensive comprehension of lobster developments, relocation examples, and collaborations with their current circumstance.

   Hut et al. (2017) featured the capability of submerged acoustic organizations in marine environment. Cooperative endeavors can upgrade the arrangement of such organizations for nonstop lobster checking, giving priceless experiences into their conduct overstretched periods.

3. **Propels in DNA Examination for Populace Hereditary qualities**

   Ecological DNA (eDNA) for Populace Studies

   Teaming up with geneticists and sub-atomic scientists, lobster observing projects can consolidate ecological DNA (eDNA) investigation for populace reviews. This creative procedure includes gathering water tests from lobster environments and breaking down the hereditary material (e.g., shed exoskeleton pieces) present in the water. This harmless methodology gives data about the overflow and variety of lobster populaces.

Thomsen et al. (2012) showed the pertinence of eDNA examination in marine conditions. Cooperative exploration can refine and grow the utilization of eDNA in lobster checking, offering a practical and productive strategy for surveying populace elements.

Genomic Devices for Figuring out Transformation

Progressions in genomic advances offer remarkable experiences into the hereditary premise of lobster transformation to changing ecological circumstances. Teaming up with geneticists and bioinformaticians, analysts can utilize genomic apparatuses to concentrate on the versatile reactions of lobster populaces to elements like temperature varieties, natural surroundings modifications, and openness to contaminations.

Jeffery et al. (2020) underlined the significance of genomics in grasping transformative cycles. Future joint efforts can dive into the genomics of lobsters, unwinding the atomic components behind their versatility and transformation despite ecological difficulties.

4. **Computerized reasoning (man-made intelligence) and AI for Information Investigation**

Robotized Picture Acknowledgment for Populace Evaluations

In a joint effort with PC researchers, lobster observing projects can execute computerized picture acknowledgment utilizing man-made brainpower (man-made intelligence) and AI (ML) calculations. This innovation empowers the examination of submerged symbolism to assess lobster overflow, size dissemination, and living space inclinations. Coordinating simulated intelligence and ML in picture handling speeds up the information examination cycle and improves the precision of populace evaluations.

Johansen et al. (2019) showed the use of computer based intelligence in marine picture examination. Future coordinated efforts can additionally refine these innovations for lobster checking, giving savvy and versatile answers for populace evaluations.

Prescient Displaying for Biological system Elements

Teaming up with information researchers, lobster observing projects can utilize prescient displaying methods to grasp the more extensive elements of seaside biological systems.

By coordinating information on lobster populaces, natural factors, and human exercises, these models can recreate future situations, assisting specialists with expecting the effect of changes and figure out proactive preservation systems.

McCarthy et al. (2018) featured the capability of prescient demonstrating in marine nature. Cooperative endeavors can use AI calculations to improve the prescient abilities of models, adding to more educated dynamic in lobster protection and the executives.

5. **Brilliant Sea Advancements for Continuous Checking**
Web of Things (IoT) Sensors in Lobster Environments
Working together with engineers and IoT subject matter experts, lobster observing projects can convey savvy sea advances furnished with sensors in lobster living spaces. These sensors can gather continuous information on natural boundaries like temperature, saltiness, and oxygen levels. Cooperative endeavors can prompt the improvement of an organized framework that gives persistent, high-recurrence information, offering a powerful perspective on lobster territory conditions.

Li et al. (2021) showed the utilization of IoT sensors in marine conditions. Future coordinated efforts can develop these innovations, making an organized framework for thorough and constant lobster observing.

Information Combination Stages for All encompassing Bits of knowledge

To expand the utility of information gathered from different sources, co-ordinated efforts with information mix experts can prompt the advancement of stages that merge and investigate assorted datasets. Coordinating data from satellite following, acoustic telemetry, eDNA examination, and natural sensors into a concentrated stage empowers specialists to acquire all encompassing experiences into lobster biology and biological system elements.

Smith et al. (2022) underlined the significance of coordinated information stages in marine exploration. Future cooperative endeavors can zero in on making easy to use, information driven stages that work with cross-disciplinary examinations and illuminate proof based direction.

6. **Difficulties and Contemplations in Embracing Arising Advances**

Interdisciplinary Coordinated effort for Innovation Reception
While arising innovations offer gigantic potential, their effective reception requires interdisciplinary joint effort. Working together with specialists from assorted fields — sea life science, designing, hereditary qualities, software engineering, and that's only the tip of the iceberg — guarantees that the execution of these advancements is logically significant, experimentally thorough, and lined up with the objectives of lobster checking programs.

Claudet et al. (2008) accentuated the meaning of successful interdisciplinary joint effort. Laying out correspondence channels, cultivating common comprehension, and advancing a common vision are fundamental contemplations in cooperative endeavors pointed toward coordinating arising advancements into lobster observing.

Information Security and Moral Contemplations

As cooperative endeavors outfit the force of trend setting innovations, tending to information security and moral contemplations becomes principal. Working together with ethicists, lawful specialists, and information protection experts guarantees that the sending of advancements follows moral norms, regards security, and shields the honesty of the information gathered.

Jones et al. (2021) highlighted the significance of moral contemplations in marine examination. Future joint efforts should focus on moral rules, straight-forwardness, and partner commitment to assemble trust and guarantee the mindful utilization of arising advancements in lobster checking.

7.2 Potential for Lobster Monitoring in Climate Change Studies

As environmental change keeps on applying its effect on marine biological systems, the job of cornerstone species, like lobsters, turns out to be progressively huge in understanding and answering ecological movements. Lobster populaces are especially delicate to changes in temperature, sea fermentation, and natural surroundings adjustments, making them important markers for environmental change studies. This investigation dives into the potential for lobster checking in environmental change studies, analyzing the bits of knowledge acquired, challenges confronted, and future headings in utilizing these notorious scavangers as sentinels of natural change.

1. **Lobsters as Environmental Change Sentinels: Bits of knowledge from Observing**

   Temperature Awareness and Warm Resilience

   Teaming up with sea life scholars, environment researchers can use lobster observing information to survey the temperature awareness and warm resistance of various lobster species. Long haul temperature records, combined with perceptions of lobster conduct and conveyance, give important bits of knowledge into how these shellfish answer varieties in water temperature.

   Hobday et al. (2016) underscored the significance of figuring out warm resilience in marine species. Lobster checking programs add to this comprehension by catching information on temperature-subordinate cycles, for example, development rates, conceptive achievement, and transient examples, supporting the expectation of how lobster populaces might adjust or change in light of environmental change.

   Sea Fermentation Effects on Lobster Physiology

   The joint effort between sea life scholars and environment researchers reaches out to concentrating on the effects of sea fermentation on lobster physiology. By breaking down the information gathered from lobster checking programs, scientists can investigate what changes in seawater science mean for parts of lobster science, including shedding, calcification, and in general wellbeing.

Mackenzie et al. (2014) featured the interconnectedness of sea fermentation and lobster physiology. Cooperative endeavors in checking projects can give pivotal information to figuring out the perplexing collaborations between natural stressors and lobster reactions, helping with the detailing of methodologies for moderating the effects of sea fermentation on these imperative shellfish.

2. **Lobster Observing and Territory Elements**
   Changes in Natural surroundings Reasonableness
   Teaming up with biologists and ecological researchers, lobster checking programs add to the appraisal of living space elements affected by environmental change. Changes in temperature and sea flows can prompt changes in the appropriation and reasonableness of lobster living spaces. By observing lobster overflow and circulation designs, specialists can distinguish regions where environment driven changes are influencing the accessibility of reasonable territories.

   Scheffer et al. (2018) underscored the significance of understanding environment elements with regards to environmental change. Lobster checking programs assume a significant part in giving observational information that illuminates expectations about how territories might move because of changing natural circumstances, considering proactive protection and the board procedures.

   Effect of Ocean Level Ascent on Beach front Environments
   Environmental change achieves rising ocean levels, which can significantly affect waterfront living spaces that lobsters occupy. Teaming up with waterfront environmentalists, analysts can use lobster observing information to evaluate the effect of ocean level ascent on the accessibility and nature of lobster territories. Understanding how these progressions impact lobster populaces is essential for creating versatile administration systems.

   IPCC (2019) featured the meaning of concentrating on the effects of ocean level ascent on seaside biological systems. Lobster checking programs, in a joint effort with specialists in ocean level ascent influences, add to the more extensive comprehension of what environmental change-prompted modifications in waterfront natural surroundings mean for the circulation and soundness of lobster populaces.

3. **Cooperative Exploration on Environment Related Stressors**
   Impacts of Outrageous Climate Occasions
   Teaming up with environment researchers, lobster observing projects contribute important information on the impacts of outrageous climate

occasions on lobster populaces. Tropical storms, heatwaves, and other outrageous occasions can affect lobster natural surroundings, food accessibility, and generally speaking environment wellbeing. The cooperative examination of observing information permits scientists to survey how these occasions impact lobster conduct, endurance rates, and conceptive achievement.

Przeslawski et al. (2015) featured the need to concentrate on the effects of outrageous occasions on marine biological systems. Lobster checking programs, as a team with environment researchers, give an extraordinary chance to catch constant reactions of lobster populaces to outrageous climate occasions, upgrading how we might interpret the strength and weaknesses of these species despite environment inconstancy.

Collaboration with Other Environment Related Stressors

Cooperative exploration reaches out to concentrating on the associations between various environment related stressors. Lobster observing projects, as a team with biologists and natural researchers, contribute information on the combined effects of variables, for example, temperature changes, sea fermentation, territory movements, and outrageous climate occasions on lobster populaces.

Harris et al. (2020) accentuated the significance of considering numerous stressors in environmental change studies. By incorporating information from different sources, cooperative endeavors can unwind the complicated transaction of stressors, giving a more thorough comprehension of what environmental change means for lobster biology.

4. **Challenges in Lobster Observing for Environmental Change Studies**
Information Inconstancy and Long haul Checking
One of the difficulties in using lobster observing information for environmental change studies is the inborn fluctuation in natural circumstances. Partners need to represent factors like normal vacillations in lobster populaces, occasional varieties, and confined influences that might veil the drawn out patterns related with environmental change.

Johnson et al. (2018) featured the significance of long haul observing to recognize normal inconstancy from environment incited changes. Cooperative exploration ought to zero in on laying out strong observing conventions that catch information overstretched periods, empowering the distinguishing proof of environment related patterns in the midst of inborn changeability.

Restricted Standard Information for Authentic Investigation
Authentic examination of environment trent prompted changes in lobster populaces is upset by the restricted accessibility of gauge information. Colleagues need to address the test of deficient authentic information to lay out exhaustive patterns. This constraint accentuates the significance of

cooperative endeavors in making review datasets through the joining of different sources, including logical studies, fishery records, and authentic information.

Chan et al. (2021) highlighted the requirement for authentic setting in environmental change studies. Cooperative examination drives can investigate ways of incorporating verifiable records with contemporary checking information, giving a more nuanced comprehension of how lobster populaces have answered environmental change over the long run.

5. **Future Headings in Lobster Observing for Environmental Change Studies**

Improving Interdisciplinary Coordinated effort

The fate of lobster checking in environmental change studies requires a significantly more grounded accentuation on interdisciplinary coordinated effort. Connecting with scientists from different fields, including environment science, sea life science, biology, hereditary qualities, and ecological checking, guarantees a comprehensive and nuanced comprehension of how lobsters answer environment prompted changes.

Palumbi et al. (2014) underlined the force of interdisciplinary cooperation in sea life science. Future drives ought to focus on cooperative examination programs that unite specialists with shifted skill, cultivating a complete way to deal with concentrating on the effects of environmental change on lobster populaces.

Consolidating Resident Science for Adaptable Information Assortment

To conquer the test of restricted information and extend observing endeavors, future joint efforts can investigate the combination of resident science drives. Drawing in people in general in lobster checking upgrades information assortment capacities as well as advances natural mindfulness and training. Partners can work with networks to lay out resident science programs that contribute significant information on lobster overflow, conduct, and natural surroundings use.

Silvertown (2009) featured the capability of resident science in biodiversity observing. Cooperative endeavors ought to consider imaginative ways of including nearby networks, fishers, and devotees in information assortment, making a greater and decentralized observing organization.

Using Trend setting innovations for Accuracy Checking

Headways in innovation offer uncommon open doors for accuracy observing of lobster populaces. Teaming up with technologists, scientists can investigate the joining of trend setting innovations like satellite labels, submerged sensors, and independent vehicles to improve the goal and extent of lobster checking endeavors. These advances can give ongoing information, taking into account dynamic and versatile reactions to environment prompted changes.

Thompson et al. (2016) showed the capability of cutting edge innovations in marine observing. Future coordinated efforts ought to zero in on integrating these advancements into lobster checking programs, extending the tool compartment accessible for concentrating on the effects of environmental change on lobster populaces.

Long haul Interest in Checking Projects

To address the test of information fluctuation and restricted verifiable records, future cooperative endeavors ought to focus on long haul interest in observing projects. Laying out supported checking endeavors that range many years guarantees the aggregation of thorough datasets that catch the nuanced reactions of lobster populaces to environmental change over the long run.

Halpern et al. (2015) underlined the significance of long haul observing in sea life science. Partners ought to advocate for supported financing and backing for observing projects, perceiving the important commitment of constant information assortment to how we might interpret environment actuated changes in lobster populaces.

7.3 Opportunities for Further Research and Development

The field of lobster observing has seen wonderful headways, giving important bits of knowledge into the science, conduct, and reactions of these marine scavangers to different natural elements. As we leave on additional innovative work tries, a large number of chances arise to extend our comprehension, refine observing procedures, and add to more viable preservation and the executives methodologies. This investigation dives into the amazing open doors for additional innovative work in lobster checking, illustrating key regions where progressions can essentially upgrade our insight and effect on these urgent parts of beach front environments.

1. **Progressing Mechanical Applications**

   Coordination of Man-made brainpower (artificial intelligence) and AI (ML)

   Open doors lie in propelling the mix of artificial intelligence and ML calculations into lobster observing cycles.

   Teaming up with PC researchers and information experts, scientists can improve the proficiency of information examination, mechanize picture acknowledgment for populace appraisals, and foster prescient models for biological system elements. This reconciliation can smooth out the understanding of complex datasets, considering speedier and more exact experiences into lobster populaces and their reactions to natural changes. Smith et al. (2022) stressed the capability of computer based intelligence and ML in marine exploration. Future examination can investigate novel uses of these advances in lobster checking, opening open doors for continuous direction and further developed asset allotment in preservation endeavors.

Joining of Web of Things (IoT) Sensors

The turn of events and organization of IoT sensors in lobster territories present energizing open doors for constant, high-recurrence information assortment. Teaming up with engineers and IoT trained professionals, specialists can lay out sensor networks that screen natural boundaries, giving constant experiences into territory conditions. This ongoing information can altogether improve how we might interpret transient vacillations and work with versatile administration techniques.

Li et al. (2021) exhibited the utilization of IoT sensors in marine conditions. Future examination can zero in on growing the utilization of these sensors in lobster observing, encouraging a dynamic and responsive way to deal with natural changes.

2. **Hereditary and Atomic Exploration**

Genomic Studies for Environment Variation Experiences

Amazing open doors have large amounts of progressing genomic studies to investigate how lobsters adjust to changing environment conditions. Teaming up with geneticists and atomic scientists, analysts can dig into the genomics of various lobster populaces to distinguish hereditary markers related with environment flexibility. This data can offer basic experiences into the versatile limit of lobsters and illuminate protection procedures that advance the tirelessness of tough populaces.

Jeffery et al. (2020) featured the significance of genomics in figuring out developmental cycles. Further exploration can disentangle the atomic components that underlie lobster reactions to environment stressors, adding to the advancement of designated preservation draws near.

Ecological DNA (eDNA) for Biodiversity Appraisal

Growing the utilization of eDNA examination gives open doors to more extensive biodiversity evaluations in lobster environments. Teaming up with sub-atomic biologists, analysts can refine eDNA strategies to recognize the presence of lobster species as well as evaluate the general biodiversity and strength of biological systems.

This approach can give an all encompassing comprehension of the natural setting in which lobsters flourish.

Thomsen et al. (2012) exhibited the relevance of eDNA examination in marine conditions. Future examination can investigate creative uses of eDNA to screen changes in local area structure, giving a more extensive viewpoint on the effects of ecological changes on lobster natural surroundings.

3. **Environmental Change Strength Studies**
Long haul Environment Versatility Appraisals
Open doors exist in leading long haul evaluations of lobster populaces to comprehend their versatility to environmental change. Working together with environment researchers and scientists, specialists can lay out observing projects that range several decades. Long haul datasets offer experiences into how lobster populaces adjust overstretched periods, giving a premise to foreseeing and overseeing future changes because of environment fluctuation.

Halpern et al. (2015) underlined the significance of long haul observing in sea life science. Further exploration drives can focus on supported endeavors, considering the distinguishing proof of patterns, transformation examples, and expected edges in lobster populaces.

Local area Based Transformation Systems
Teaming up with networks and social researchers presents open doors for creating local area based transformation methodologies. Drawing in nearby occupants in the co-formation of versatile measures guarantees that methodologies are logically important, upgrade local area strength, and encourage feasible jobs. This approach recognizes the significance of consolidating nearby information and values in environment transformation endeavors.

Adger et al. (2005) featured the job of networks in transformation systems. Future examination can investigate ways of coordinating conventional natural information with logical experiences, encouraging a cooperative methodology that lines up with the financial setting of beach front networks.

4. **Upgraded Territory Planning and Checking**
High-Goal Satellite Symbolism for Definite Territory Planning
Open doors lie in propelling the utilization of high-goal satellite symbolism for definite territory planning. Teaming up with remote detecting subject matter experts, specialists can outfit the force of cutting edge satellite advancements to make exact guides of lobster territories. This degree of detail empowers a more nuanced comprehension of the particular ecological highlights that impact lobster circulation and overflow.

Turner et al. (2015) featured the capability of high-goal satellite symbolism in environment observing. Future exploration can zero in on refining and growing these advances to add to living space protection and the executives methodologies custom-made to the particular requirements of lobster populaces.

Submerged Acoustic Checking Organizations for Ceaseless Perception
Growing the utilization of submerged acoustic checking networks expresses open doors for ceaseless viewpoint of lobster conduct. Teaming

up with acoustics specialists and innovation engineers, scientists can lay out organizations of submerged beneficiaries that give constant information on lobster developments, collaborations, and reactions to ecological changes. This persistent perception improves the fleeting goal of checking endeavors, catching powerful environmental cycles.

Cabin et al. (2017) featured the capability of submerged acoustic organizations in marine nature. Further exploration can investigate the adaptability and materialness of these organizations in various lobster living spaces, giving significant experiences into fine-scale standards of conduct.

5. **Resident Science Commitment**

Versatile Applications for Resident Science Investment

Amazing open doors exist in creating and using versatile applications to upgrade resident science cooperation in lobster observing. Teaming up with programming engineers and teachers, specialists can plan easy to understand applications that engage residents to add to information assortment endeavors. These applications can work with the detailing of lobster perceptions, screen waterfront conditions, and draw in a more extensive crowd in logical undertakings.

Dickinson et al. (2012) focused on the capability of versatile applications in resident science. Future examination can investigate imaginative ways of utilizing innovation for resident commitment, making a more comprehensive and broad organization of supporters of lobster observing projects.

Local area Researcher Cooperation for Information Assortment

The cooperation among researchers and nearby networks in information assortment offers remarkable open doors for increasing observing endeavors. Connecting with local area individuals as dynamic members in observing projects upgrades information assortment capacities as well as cultivates a feeling of responsibility and stewardship. Partners can work intimately with networks to foster conventions, give preparing, and lay out criticism systems for powerful cooperation.

Silvertown (2009) underlined the capability of resident science in biodiversity checking. Future exploration can investigate models of local area researcher cooperation that are socially delicate, enabling, and add to a mutual perspective of lobster environment.

6. **Interdisciplinary Methodologies**

Social-Biological Frameworks Exploration for Comprehensive Getting it

Valuable open doors exist in propelling social-natural frameworks examination to accomplish a more all encompassing comprehension of lobster environment. Working together with sociologists, anthropologists, and market analysts, scientists can investigate the unpredictable associations between human exercises and lobster populaces. This approach considers the financial components of lobster fisheries, the effect of the board strategies, and the social meaning of lobsters to nearby networks.

Berkes et al. (2003) featured the significance of social-biological frameworks research. Further examination can incorporate social and biological viewpoints, giving an extensive structure to leaders to foster reasonable and versatile administration systems.

Reconciliation with Other Observing Methodologies

Teaming up with analysts from other observing disciplines presents open doors for mix and cooperative energy. Joining lobster observing information with data from other marine species, water quality evaluations, and biological system wellbeing markers can give a more extensive comprehension of beach front environments. This interdisciplinary methodology encourages co-operation across logical spaces and improves the ability to address complex biological difficulties.

Levin et al. (2017) accentuated the worth of coordinated observing methodologies. Future examination can investigate instruments for cross-disciplinary joint effort, creating structures that empower the consistent mix of assorted observing datasets.